GOOD NEWS ABOUT WOMEN & HPV

ALEXANDER MORTAKIS MD, PhD

GOOD NEWS ABOUT WOMEN & HPV

Find out how to protect your health,
the health of your children,
and your relationship with your partner.

ΕΚΔΟΣΕΙΣ ΠΑΤΑΚΗ

To my patients, the women who have honored me with their trust, who have inspired and taught me

CONTENTS

Preface by Silvia de Sanjosé 33
Preface by Jacob Bornstein 37
Author's note 39
Acknowledgments 45

CHAPTER 1
HPV infections and potential outcomes

HPV: What it is, where it is and what it causes

1. What does HPV mean? 48
2. Is it a single virus? 48
3. What does HPV cause? 49
4. Where do we find HPV? 49
5. On what areas of the human body does HPV live and multiply? 49
6. What are papillomas and what are condylomas? 51

HPV: Not all types of HPV are the same. Which ones may lead to cancer?

7. Genital types of HPV: What areas do they infect andwhat do they cause? 52
8. Genital types of HPV: Is the specific type important? Are they all dangerous? 54
9. Low-risk types of HPV: what do they cause? 54
10. High-risk types of HPV: what do they cause? 55

What can happen to you after the infection?

11. How does HPV multiply in your cells?........... 57
12. If infected, is a lesion certain to occur? 60
13. What kinds of lesions may appear in the near future, following the infection?................... 61
14. If you are infected today, when will the first lesions appear?............................... 63
15. What happens after genital warts appear? 63
16. Are genital warts life-threatening? 63
17. If you have invisible (subclinical) lesions from HPV on the cervix at this time, how can you know about it? 63
18. Are you at direct risk from the invisible lesions caused immediately after the infection?........ 64

How and when will HPV infection lead to cancer?

19. How can HPV drive your cells crazy? 64
20. What is the most frequent cancer in women caused by HPV?....................... 65
21. Which women are at a higher risk for cervical cancer?............................... 66
22. If a woman is infected with an oncogenic type of HPV, will cervical cancer develop immediately?........................... 66
23. Why is cervical cancer considered preventable?..... 66
24. How can a woman know that she is not at risk? 67
25. In what organs, other than the cervix, can high-risk types of HPV cause cancer? 67
26. How can doctors tell the difference between premalignant lesions and simple infections?..... 68
27. What are LSIL and HSIL?................... 68

Genital types of HPV: How are they transmitted?

28. Where is the HPV that will infect you located? 69
29. How are genital types of HPV transmitted? 69

Oncogenic types of HPV: Sneaky invaders - Dangerous roommates. What can you do?

30. Can you know if you have been infected in the past by an oncogenic type of HPV or if you have an active infection in your cervical cells right now?. 72
31. If an HPV infection is suppressed, does the risk continue to exist? 72
32. Does HPV ever leave your body? Do you have to keep having check-ups?. 73
33. How can HPV appear again after many years? 73
34. Once with HPV – always with HPV?. 73
35. How do you explain that many people are infected by HPV viruses but only a few have serious problems from them? .... .74
36. How can a woman know that she is not at risk? 75

What are your chances of becoming infected by genital types of HPV?

37. How frequent are HPV infections in the population?. 75
38. Does the chance of infection by genital types of HPV increase depending on the number of sexual partners?. 76
39. What is the probability of becoming infected by a new partner?. 76
40. Can you know if your partner has an active infection at this time? 78

41. Are there high-risk sexual partners?............ 78
42. What is the possibility of a person becoming
    infected by HPV over his or her lifetime?....... 78
43. Does the use of a condom prevent HPV infection?... 79

What can you do to protect your health?

44. What does prevention include?................ 80
45. What is primary prevention?.................. 80
46. What is secondary prevention?................ 80

CHAPTER 2
Prevention of infection from specific types of HPV with vaccination

47. Which vaccines have been made available to date? .. 84
48. How do vaccines against HPV work? 84
49. Do the vaccines prevent against all types of HPV?. . . 85
50. Which types of HPV do vaccines protect you from?. . 85
51. Which HPV-related diseases do the vaccines protect you from? 86
52. How was the effectiveness of the vaccines proven?. . . 87
53. What about head and neck cancers attributed to HPV? 88
54. Do the vaccines contain viruses? 89
55. Are vaccines a method of prevention or a method of treatment? 89
56. Should boys be vaccinated? 89
57. What is the ideal age for vaccination? 90
58. Is vaccination recommended even after the beginning of sexual activity? 91
59. How is the vaccine administered? Trends and most recent estimates 91
60. How safe are the vaccines? 92
61. What are the side effects of the vaccines? 92
62. Indications for the new Gardasil 9. 93
63. What do we know about the vaccine during pregnancy? 94
64. What happens if a woman becomes pregnant before completing the three doses? 94
65. After they are vaccinated, should women continue to have check-ups? 94
66. Is there a therapeutic vaccine for HPV? 94
67. Do vaccines lead to increased sexual activity in young people? 94
68. Is an HPV DNA test recommended before the vaccination? 95

CHAPTER 3
HPV and the female lower genital tract

Why are check-ups necessary?

69. In what areas of the female genital organs does HPV cause cancer?............................ 98
70. Why cervical cancer caused by HPV should not worry you if you have regular check-ups............ 98
71. How long does it take for a precancerous lesion to form?................................ 99
72. If there are any precancerous lesions, what would be the symptoms?........................ 99
73. Are precancerous lesions visible during a gynecological examination? How are they discovered?....... 99
74. Why should lesions be found while they are still invisible to the naked eye?.................100

HPV hides in the cervix...

75. In what type of cervical cells does HPV cause cancer?............................101
76. How do we find precancerous lesions in the cervix?............................103

CONTENTS

CHAPTER 4
Pap test

PAP TEST

77. What is the Pap test?........................107
78. How is the Pap test performed?...............107
79. What do we mean by a negative Pap test?........107
80. Can a Pap test come out negative and miss a lesion?...............................107
81. Is it possible to have more serious lesions than what the Pap test showed?.................108
82. What is the reliability of the Pap test?...........108
83. How can the reliability of the Pap test be improved?..............................109
84. What can the examination of the cervical cells under the microscope show?...............109
85. If the Pap test shows inflammation or atrophy, what happens next?......................110
86. If the Pap test shows abnormal cells, what is their significance and what are the next steps to be taken?...................................110
87. Is any preparation necessary before a Pap test?.....113
88. At what age should women start getting Pap tests?..113
89. Up to what age should women keep getting Pap tests?............................114
90. Should women get Pap tests during pregnancy?....114
91. Must women who are not sexually active at present have a Pap test?.........................115
92. Must women who have had a hysterectomy get Pap tests?...............................115

CHAPTER 5
HPV test

93. What is the HPV test? 118
94. What is the logic behind the HPV test? 118
95. How is the HPV test performed? 118
96. Can an HPV test be performed together with
     the Pap test? 118
97. At what age is it recommended that women get
     an HPV test and why? 119
98. If the HPV test comes out positive, does this mean
     that you have something serious? 120
99. What is the reliability of the HPV test and the double
     test? 120
100. How should a woman prepare before an HPV test? . . 120
101. Are there HPV tests that show the type
     of the virus? 120
102. Are there different types of HPV tests? 120
103. What are the possible results of the HPV test
     and what do they mean? 121
104. In what cases in general are HPV tests
     recommended? 121

CHAPTER 6
Colposcopy – Biopsy

Colposcopy

105. What is a colposcope?......................124
106. What is a colposcopy?......................124
107. What is the colposcopy used for?..............125
108. Is the colposcope used during surgery?..........125
109. When is a colposcopy recommended?...........126
110. How is the colposcopy performed?.............126
111. Are biopsies always performed during
     a colposcopy?...........................126
112. Are the colposcopy and biopsies painful?........127
113. Does the colposcopy have any risk?.............127
114. Can you get a colposcopy during pregnancy?......127
115. Is any preparation necessary before a colposcopy?...127
116. How reliable is a colposcopy?.................128

Colposcopic biopsy

117. What exactly is a colposcopic biopsy and how is it
     performed?.............................128
118. Why do we perform biopsies?.................128
119. What is the reliability of a biopsy during
     a colposcopy?...........................129
120. What does the doctor see under the microscope
     when examining a biopsy?..................130
121. What is the difference between a biopsy and
     a Pap test?.............................130
122. What are the possible diagnoses after a cervical
     biopsy?...............................130
123. How do we get from a check-up to a biopsy?......131

CHAPTER 7
Benign diseases caused by genital types of HPV

Subclinical lesions on the skin and mucous membranes

124. What are subclinical lesions caused by HPV?......134
125. How frequent are subclinical lesions caused by HPV?...............................134
126. What is the incidence of subclinical lesions caused by HPV in the general population compared to the incidence of genital warts?............134
127. Do subclinical lesions cause symptoms? How are they discovered?.......................135
128. What types of HPV cause subclinical lesions?......135
129. What is the prognosis for subclinical lesions caused by HPV?...............................135
130. If an infection by a cancer-causing type of HPV is discovered, what is the next step?..........136
131. What is the treatment for subclinical lesions?......136
132. Which subclinical lesions do we follow up and why?...............................136

Genital warts

A) What are genital warts, what causes them and how will you recognize them?

133. What are genital warts?....................136
134. What causes genital warts?..................136
135. What do genital warts look like?...............137
136. Is it a common disease?....................137
137. Where do warts appear in women?.............137
138. Where do warts appear in men?...............138
139. Is the appearance of warts in the mouth frequent? ..139
140. What types of HPV cause genital warts?.........139

CONTENTS

B) Transmission of genital warts
141. How are genital warts transmitted?.............139
142. If you have intercourse with an infected individual, is infection inevitable?....................140
143. How long after the infection do genital warts appear?..............................141
144. How can you know if the individual you will have intercourse with has the infection and that you may become infected?....................142
145. What are your chances of contracting genital warts from a partner?.......................142
146. How can you find out when and who infected you?...143
147. If someone has common warts, can they infect you with genital warts?......................143
148. How can we explain genital warts in areas where there is no friction during sexual intercourse?...143
149. If a woman gets genital warts, must her partner be examined?..........................143

C) Diagnosis of genital warts
150. What are the symptoms of genital warts?..........144
151. How does a woman discover genital warts?.......144
152. How can you know if you have genital warts elsewhere?.............................144
153. What is the association between genital warts and cancers caused by HPV?...............144
154. What tests should you get if you develop genital warts?................................145
155. Can a woman with genital warts get a negative HPV test?............................145

D) Treatment of genital warts
156. Can genital warts and HPV infection be treated?....145
157. What are the treatments for genital warts?........145

158. What medications or substances are used to treat genital warts?................................146
159. How are genital warts destroyed?..............148
160. When and how are warts removed?............150
161. Which is the best treatment for genital warts?......150
162. Do genital warts recur after treatment?..........150
163. How is the recurrence of genital warts after treatment explained?............................150
164. How can you increase the treatment's success rates? . 151

E) Prevention of genital warts
165. Is there a way to prevent genital warts?..........152
166. How can you protect yourself?................152
167. What should you do to avoid infecting others?.....152
168. Is there any point in getting vaccinated if you have ever had genital warts in the past?..............153

Recurring respiratory papillomatosis

169. What is respiratory papillomatosis?.............153
170. At what ages does it appear and how common is it? .153
171. What is the cause of respiratory papillomatosis?....154
172. What are the symptoms?....................154
173. How is it diagnosed?.......................155
174. How is it treated?..........................155
175. What is the prognosis?.....................155
176. Is there any prevention?....................155

CHAPTER 8
Precancerous lesions on the cervix

From infection to precancerous lesions and cancer

177. What is the cause of cervical cancer?............158
178. How can HPV cause cancer?..................158
179. What do the terms LSIL and HSIL of the cervix
     mean?................................159
180. What are CIN1, CIN2, and CIN3? 162
181. What is the prognosis for CIN1, CIN2,
     and CIN3/CIS?........................162
182. Which terms are used internationally
     for precancerous lesions on the cervix?........163

What does the diagnosis involve?

183. Are cervical precancerous lesions visible during
     a gynecological examination? How are they
     discovered?...........................165
184. Why should lesions be found when they are still
     invisible to the naked eye examination?........165
185. What are the necessary tests and in what order
     should they be performed? 166

Treatment of cervical precancerous lesions

186. What is the purpose of the treatment?...........166
187. What treatments are there available?............167
188. How is the most appropriate method selected? 167
189. What are the criteria used to choose the correct
     treatment for the lesions?..................168
190. What happens if HSIL or CIN2/3 lesions
     are discovered during pregnancy? 169

Description of procedures

191. What is the logic behind these procedures? 169
192. What should the patient do to prepare before
     the procedure?. 171

LEEP

193. What does it mean? 171
194. Does the LEEP procedure require anesthesia? 172
195. How is the procedure performed?. 172
196. What are the complications and risks of a LEEP
     procedure? 173
197. Post-operative instructions. 174
198. What are the future risks after a LEEP procedure?. . . 175

COLD-KNIFE CONIZATION

199. What is it?. 175
200. When is it performed?. 176
201. How is the procedure performed?. 176
202. What are the procedure's risks? 176

LASER CONIZATION

203. What is it and what are its advantages? 177
204. In which cases is it preferred? 178
205. What are its complications? 178

Procedures that destroy the transformation zone

LASER ABLATION OF THE TRANSFORMATION ZONE

206. What is it and how is it done? 179
207. What are the advantages and disadvantages
     of the method?. 179

CRYOTHERAPY

208. How is it done?........................180
209. What are the advantages and disadvantages of the method?............................180

Post-operative follow-up and recurrences

210. Is follow-up necessary after the lesions are treated?..181
211. Will you be transmitting the HPV infection after treatment?..........................182
212. If you get treatment and the HPV lesions are gone, is there a risk of becoming reinfected by your partner?............................182

CHAPTER 9
Precancerous lesions caused by HPV in the vagina, vulva, and anus

Vaginal precancerous lesions (VaIN)

213. What are VaINs? 184
214. How are they diagnosed? 184
215. Which lesions require treatment? 185
216. How are high-grade lesions (HSIL/VaIN2, 3) treated? 185
217. Can vaginal precancerous lesions appear in women who have had their uterus removed? 185
218. What is the effect of smoking on VaIN lesions? 186

HPV-related precancerous lesions of the vulva (VIN)

219. What does VIN mean? 187
220. How are HPV-related VIN lesions classified? 187
221. Are HPV-related VIN lesions visible? 187
222. How are the lesions diagnosed? 188
223. How are HPV-related VIN lesions treated? 188
224. What does treatment entail and what are the criteria? 188
225. Do the lesions recur after treatment? Is follow-up necessary? 189

Precancerous lesions of the anal canal (AIN) and the perianal area (PaIN)

226. What are AIN lesions? 189
227. How are AIN lesions classified? 190
228. What is the prognosis for AIN lesions? 191
229. What are PaIN lesions and how can they be classified? 191

230. Who is at risk for AIN and PaIN?..............191
231. What preventive measures are recommended?......192
232. Are there symptoms from the AIN/PaIN lesions?...192
233. How are the lesions diagnosed?...............192
234. How are AIN/PaIN lesions treated?............193
235. Which AIN lesions require treatment?..........193
236. How are high-grade lesions (HSIL/AIN2, 3) treated?............................193
237. Do AIN and PaIN lesions recur after treatment? Is follow-up necessary?...................194
238. How frequent are HSIL/AIN2, 3 lesions in the general population?..........................194
239. Are women with high-grade lesions (HSIL) in an organ at an increased risk for similar lesions in other organs?...................194

CHAPTER 10
Cancers caused by genital types of HPV

240. What is cancer? 196
241. In which organs do genital types of HPV
cause cancer? 197
242. Does HPV cause all the cancers in the above
organs? 197
243. Other than an oncogenic type of HPV, are there
other factors that lead to carcinogenesis? 198

Cervical cancer

244. What is the frequency of cervical cancer? 200
245. Which types of HPV cause cervical cancer more
frequently? 200
246. At what age does it usually affect women? 200
247. Which women are at a higher risk for cervical
cancer? 201
248. Does cervical cancer develop overnight? 201
249. What are the symptoms of cervical cancer? 201
250. How is a cervical cancer diagnosis made? 202
251. What is staging? 202
252. What is metastasis? 204
253. What are the treatments for cervical cancer? 205
254. What is the prognosis for invasive cervical
cancer? 205
255. How successful is the prevention of cervical
cancer? 205

HPV-related vaginal cancer

256. How common is vaginal cancer? 206
257. Is HPV the cause of vaginal cancer? 206

258. Which women are at a higher risk for vaginal
     cancer? 206
259. What about vaginal cancer prevention measures? .. 206
260. What is the treatment of vaginal cancer? 207

HPV-related vulvar cancer

261. How common is vulvar cancer? 208
262. What percentage of vulvar cancers is attributed to
     oncogenic types of HPV?................. 208
263. What factors increase the chance of HPV-related
     vulvar cancer?....................... 208
264. What are the symptoms, what does it look like? ... 209
265. What does diagnosis entail?................ 209
266. What happens after the initial biopsy?.......... 209
267. How is vulvar cancer treated?............... 209
268. Why should VIN lesions be found and treated? 210
269. Can HPV-related vulvar cancers be prevented?..... 210

Anal cancer

270. What is the cause of anal cancer? 211
271. How common is anal cancer?................. 211
272. At what age does anal cancer usually appear?...... 211
273. What are the signs and symptoms of anal cancer?... 211
274. What is the connection between anal warts
     and anal cancer? 212
275. What tests are recommended for the prevention
     of anal cancer?........................ 213
276. Can anal cancer be prevented? 213

Head and neck cancer attributed to HPV

277. What are the factors for carcinogenesis in the head
     and neck? 214

278. Where do HPV-related cancers usually appear? 214
279. How is HPV transmitted to the oropharynx? 214
280. How common are oropharyngeal HPV infections?. . . 215
281. Does HPV cause carcinogenesis in the oropharynx
     immediately after the infection? 215
282. At what ages does oropharyngeal cancer appear? . . . 216
283. Should a couple's sex life change if an oropharyngeal
     HPV lesion is discovered? 216
284. What prevention measures can be taken
     for oropharyngeal cancer? 216
285. Is there any test that finds lesions? 216
286. How can you find out if you should be concerned
     about any symptom you are experiencing?. 217

CHAPTER 11
Men and HPV
(everything your partner would like to know)

Transmission of the infection and effects on men

287. How common are infections from genital types
of HPV in men?...................... 220
288. How are genital types of HPV transmitted in men?. 220
289. What do genital types of HPV cause in men?..... 220
290. Which factors affect the risk of a man getting
infected by HPV?.......................224

Diagnosis and treatment

291. What are the symptoms of a man recently infected
with HPV?............................. 225
292. How are genital warts diagnosed?..............225
293. How are subclinical infections and precancerous
lesions diagnosed?......................225
294. Can a man be tested to find out if he has been
infected with HPV in the past?............. 226
295. What treatment should men get?...............227

Prevention

296. Is there any preventive test for penile cancer in men? .227
297. Is there any preventive test for anal cancer in men?. .228
298. Can an HPV infection be prevented in men?.......229

Answers to the questions of the male partner

299. Should the partner of a woman who was found
with HPV infection be checked?............ 230
300. My partner was diagnosed with an HPV infection.
What are the risks for my health?.......... 230

CHAPTER 12
You and HPV – You don't need to worry if...

The effects from genital types of HPV in you and your children

301. What are the general problems in the population?. . . .234
302. What are the psychological consequences when a woman finds out she has been infected? 234
303. What questions do couples have after a positive diagnosis of an HPV infection? What should the doctor do? 235

Don't feel bad – Overcome your fears – Be informed – Knowledge is power!

304. Is there any reason to feel bad because your doctor told you that you have been infected with HPV? 235
305. What basic knowledge must every woman have?. . . 236
306. What should you do to protect your children? 238
307. You were diagnosed with an HPV infection. Is there any risk of infecting your children?. . . . 238
308. How should you manage an HPV infection together with your partner? 238

Boost your defense mechanisms with a healthy lifestyle

309. What is the role of your defense mechanisms in carcinogenesis?. 240
310. What can you do to improve your immune system?. 241
311. Why is it good not to smoke? 241

CONTENTS

Afterword. *243*
Bibliography *247*
Glossary. *255*
Index *261*

WARNING!

This publication and the information contained in this book under no circumstances can – or intend to – serve as a substitute for medical services or provide guidance for diagnosis or treatment.

The intention of this book is exclusively informational, and in no case can it take the place of your physician's advice.

The book contains general information based on current scientific data. The case of each patient, however, is unique, and only your doctor that will examine you, and knows your history, can guide you toward the solution for your problem.

Preface by Silvia de Sanjosé, MD PhD
President of the International Papillomavirus Society

When Dr. Alexander Mortakis asked me to read his book *Good news about women and HPV*, I was immediately fascinated by the title: its directness and positive message promised a good read. I was not disappointed. Through its 12 chapters, readers can acquire a state-of-the-art knowledge about Human Papilloma Virus (HPV) and related diseases through a natural and easy-going language.

Papillomavirus are widespread in nature and infect many animals and humans. We are all likely to be exposed to them as they live in the human skin and in our mucosa. As humans, we have always evolved surrounded by HPV, and thus their presence in our bodies does not imply that we are sick. There are few of them that we worry about because if they persist in our body they may cause disease. This book is all about understanding the impact of these few viruses and how to prevent, treat, and control them. The information provided is relevant for both men and women as we know that any sexually active person is susceptible to infection by HPV and that about 5% of all human cancers are caused by a few HPV types. But there is also very good news that you will be able to learn about going through the different chapters of this book. You will learn how they can be stopped from causing problems!

The contents of the book are organized as a series of questions that many women ask their doctor or themselves. This list is thorough and covers a wide spectrum of issues that can cause unnecessary anxiety, fear, and family trouble if they are not properly answered.

The book goes through the natural history of HPV infections and disentangles the differences between less aggressive HPV types, called low risk types, and those considered more dangerous viruses, so called high risk or oncogenic types. Primary prevention through vaccination is a main chapter that explains the importance of HPV vaccines and the possibilities of reducing the burden of disease when vaccines are applied to the general population. Secondary prevention through screening is explained in a comprehensive and clear manner. This refers to the procedures commonly recommended, such as the Pap smear test and the HPV test. Women who will need further clinical evaluation will also find relevant information on what is meant by a colposcopy exam or a biopsy. The provided explanations will help allay the fears of women having to go through these tests. The book also approaches benign HPV-related diseases, such as genital warts or respiratory papillomatosis. These are diseases that may not threaten life, but will often require continuous treatment because of common relapses.

After a series of questions and answers about cancer and cancer treatment, the last chapter makes a major statement: "Overcome your fears. Be informed. Knowledge is power!" I profoundly agree with this. Those of us who have been working in this field for many years and who have provided scientific evidence for the development of new screening tests and vaccines, have lived the frustration generated by the lack of education, the lack of understanding and the confusion about its prevention. The HPV field has been, and is, a major area of research. The enormous research efforts coming from both public and private arenas have generated one of the best prophylactic vaccines ever produced. We are now seeing an enormous impact on those countries where HPV vaccination has been massively implemented in girls and young women. Also, we are now able to detect pre-neoplasic lesions in women using tools that require fewer gynecological exams while providing a more refined and accurate diagnosis.

All this knowledge will not generate the expected health benefits if it is not well understood and applied. We do need to enforce these prevention interventions on the most vulnerable populations. These include women living in poor resource settings, or marginal groups with poor access to medical care. The interventions need to be done in an affordable and sustainable way. In richer settings, where women have the ability to access many prevention and diagnostic strategies, we also need to guarantee that we do no harm. We need to adequately base our provision of health interventions on scientific knowledge. This consideration needs to reach any woman who is or has been sexually active. Not only do we need well-informed professionals, we also need our population to be knowledgeable enough to make mature decisions. When dealing with cervical cancer prevention, well-informed women will understand better why they need to have a periodic visit. By empowering them through education they will be able to request the best possible attention. Well-informed women will be more likely to better protect their health and that of her family. However, this knowledge should not be restricted to women. Men are also part of the story and can play a major role in reducing HPV infection in the population. When HPV vaccine is offered to boys and young men, the impact on the population is enormous. Although resources are not always available, we expect that in the near future our young generations will be universally vaccinated.

Dr. Mortakis' book is an example of how professional knowledge can be transferred to our families. I hope you will enjoy reading it as much as I did.

Silvia de Sanjosé, MD PhD

President of the International Papillomavirus Society
Head of the Cancer Epidemiology Research Program
at the Catalan Institute of Oncology, Spain

Preface by Professor Jacob Bornstein, MD, MPA

The book: *Good News about Women & HPV*, edited by Dr. Alexander Mortakis, is an important and timely publication that aims at informing readers about infection by papillomaviruses. In recent years, the role of HPV in the causation of benign, premalignant, and malignant conditions in men and women has been repeatedly discussed. A Nobel Prize was dedicated to the association between HPV types 16 and 18 and cancer of the cervix, and a vaccine to prevent infection by several HPV types has been produced.

However, these developments have led to confusion and even concern. Once the word "cancer" is mentioned in association with HPV, each time an HPV infection is suspected or diagnosed in a partner or a family member, concerns are raised, sometimes causing considerable anxiety and distress.

This is exactly what motivated Dr. Alexander Mortakis to write this book. He states in his introduction: "it (the book) will relieve women of any useless anxiety and help them correctly protect their health."

The book contains answers to 311 questions. This "question and answer" format makes it easy for readers to find the proper response to their problem or concern. The medical terms are explained, and the reading is easy.

This is not the first book that Dr. Mortakis has published. So far, his books targeted specialists, detailing the scientific basis of HPV infections and associated tumors. The present book, dedicated to the general public, is based on the vast knowledge that Dr. Alexander Mortakis has gained over the years and his many years of experience diagnosing and treating patients with HPV disease in his clinic.

Dr. Alexander Mortakis was trained in the universities of Athens and California and is recognized internationally as an expert in the field of HPV and Lower Genital Tract Disease.

It is my hope that this book will be a useful guide to HPV infections and will reduce the unnecessary confusion and anxiety that are associated with this infection.

Professor Jacob Bornstein, MD, MPA.
Chairman, Department of Obstetrics & Gynecology,
Galilee Medical Center – Nahariya, Israel.
Associate Dean, Bar-Ilan University Faculty of Medicine.
Chairman, Terminology Committees of the International Society for the Study of Vulvovaginal Disease (ISSVD) and of the International Federation of Colposcopy and Cervical Pathology (IFCPC).
Past President, ISSVD.

AUTHOR'S NOTE

Over the years, my patients have come to me very anxious, persistently seeking information about a subject that is of great interest to the modern woman, the Human Papilloma Virus (HPV), and the cancer risk which HPV infection entails. The women who come to see me for the first time with this subject on their mind tell me that the information they have found on the internet is confusing and that they would like some clarifications.

HPV (Human Papilloma Virus): how it becomes part of a woman's life

Let's take the example of a healthy woman who is visiting her gynecologist for her annual check-up. The doctor examines her and assures her that everything looks good. He lets her know that he has collected cells from her cervix for a Pap test and the results will be out in a week. A week later, the doctor calls her about the Pap test results. He tells her that the cells of her uterus were found to be infected with the human papilloma virus (HPV). He tells her that the test showed abnormal cells, which may even be precancerous...

Another healthy woman goes to the doctor because she noticed "a growth" on the skin of her genitalia. The doctor examines her and tells her it's a genital wart, caused by a virus called HPV (Human Papilloma Virus).

Once the words "HPV," "Pap test showing abnormal cells," and "genital warts" come out of the doctor's mouth, any woman becomes concerned. She remembers she has heard about the genital wart viruses, which can cause cancer of the womb and other cancers. She remembers she has heard something about a vaccine, but has not gotten it.

There is nothing that worries people more than to suddenly be informed that something has gone wrong with their health; something they were not aware of up to that time.

Usually, women who learn that they have been infected with HPV, ask their doctor many questions. The dialogue usually goes as follows:

– Is it serious?
– I cannot know. We must check it.
– But when you examined me last week you told me there is nothing wrong.
– Yes, because the abnormal cells seen by the Pap test are not visible during a gynecological examination.
– What are these abnormal cells? Do I have cancer?
– No, don't worry, we'll see. You must get a colposcopy, and a biopsy may be required.
– Biopsy... The word biopsy sounds bad. You said I have a virus, called HPV. Is this the virus that causes cancer, the one the vaccine came out for?
– Yes, but we don't know if you have been infected by any of the cancer-causing types of the virus or if it has caused anything serious. We must check it.

– And where did I catch the HPV virus? I don't remember ever having anything wrong with me. How is it transmitted?
– Usually through sexual intercourse.
– As far as I know, my husband never had anything, and neither did I. Is he hiding something from me?
– I cannot know, is the doctor's awkward reply.
– Can this virus be cured?
– The virus is not cured, but if it has caused precancerous lesions they can be removed.
– Precancerous lesions? Oh my God! And if I get treated, won't my husband reinfect me?
– The virus will remain in your body in any case, even after we remove the lesions, whether you have sex with your husband again or not.
– Will a virus that causes cancer stay in me forever?
– We will keep an eye on you, don't worry!

How can one describe the psychological condition of a woman being informed for the first time about something so critically related to her health? This "don't worry" is not always convincing.

The anxiety which the patient experiences is great. Many negative feelings start surfacing:
- Fear of possible cancer.
- Despair, since she cannot permanently rid herself of a virus that causes cancer.
- Remorse and guilt about her relationship with the person who transmitted this dangerous HPV, suspicion of her partner having an affair.

Conversations such as the above between patient and doctor are very frequent. Women are desperately trying to find answers to their questions.

Scientific information is invaluable

Every day, for the past thirty years, I have seen the concern, fear, and even despair in the eyes of the women sitting before me.

However, fear and panic are not the best advisors.

You are not alone in worrying about the infection, but if you get the right information, you will stop worrying. This is the reason why I wrote this book.

The book you are holding in your hands was written to provide answers to the main questions:
- Where do we stand today?
- What do we know about the diseases caused by the Human Papilloma Viruses (HPVs)?
- Are fear and panic justified?
- Are the modern woman and her daughter at risk from HPVs?
- How are HPV-related diseased prevented?
- How are HPV-related diseases diagnosed and treated?

When you read this book, you will be convinced that there is no reason for panic. The modern woman does not need to worry about herself or her children if she faithfully follows the instructions on prevention.

The medical community today takes pride in the fact that there are prevention methods available for such a major problem. There is both prevention of the infection with vaccination, and a way to prevent most cancers by detecting precancerous lesions in time and treating them.

As doctors, we know that women continue to die of HPV-related cancers, when most of them are preventable!

An informed woman who takes the proper precaution measures is not at risk. But it is not enough that we know it, it is our duty to inform women. Women need to understand how they can get HPV and how HPV can cause potentially fatal diseases. They need to know how to protect themselves.

As I mentioned above, the publication of this book is part of this effort. This book is designed to give you the knowledge you'll need to make intelligent choices.

How can you benefit from the book you are holding in your hands?

The book is separated into twelve chapters. The first six chapters present general knowledge that is useful to all women who want to learn how to protect their health and the health of their children.

The first chapter makes detailed reference to infection by HPV and the consequences such an infection may have on a woman's health (what you need to know first).

The second chapter is dedicated to the available vaccines. Detailed information is provided regarding the indications, effectiveness, and side-effects of each vaccine.

Chapters 3, 4, 5, and 6 provide detailed information regarding routine check-ups in order to diagnose in time precancerous lesions caused by HPV.

Chapters 7, 8, 9, and 10 refer to the diseases which genital types of HPV may cause to women and men. These chapters are obviously of more interest to women who are already infected and want to know more details about the risks.

Finally, the last two chapters, 11 and 12, focus on informing the couple. Almost always, after diagnosis of the infection, the couple has questions and their relationship may be affected if they are not given the proper information. An effort is made to answer the questions that cause the most anxiety for women and men. These two chapters offer some advice on how to live with HPV, how to talk to your sexual partner about HPV, and how to decrease the risks.

The book follows a question–and–answer format. Answers are given to 311 questions in total. I tried to include the most frequent questions I am asked by my patients on a daily basis. The information you will read is provided in a logical sequence so that there are no questions left as you move along in the book. You can easily search the contents and find a specific question that interests you in order to then find the answer you want. Because you may choose to find answers to specific questions without reading the book from cover to cover, it was considered necessary to repeat certain things many times. In several cases you will find references to other points of the book in order to better understand certain issues.

I wrote this book with great joy, believing that it will relieve you of any useless anxiety and help you correctly protect your health.

ACKNOWLEDGMENTS

I would first and foremost like to warmly thank my patients, the women who trusted me with their life and the life of their children.

I would also like to express my gratitude to the countless researchers – in the field of HPV-related diseases – because, thanks to their scientific work, we are today at a point where we can effectively protect and assure the health of our patients.

I would also like to thank Patakis Publications for the excellent copy-editing of the book, and I would especially like to thank Ms Elena Pataki, without whose warm encouragement this publication would not have been possible, for her assistance and advice throughout all the phases of the book's preparation. My sincere thanks to Ms Yvoni Karydi for editing the publication, and Ms Niki Antonakopoulou for desktop publishing. A big thank you to Ms Renia Metallinou, who willingly dedicated many hours to our repeated meetings in order to learn about the subject and correctly render the book's illustrations.

Finally, I would like to express my gratitude to my wife Sofia and my children Despina, Anastasia, and Stratis, for the support during the writing of the book and the understanding they showed for my countless hours of absence.

CHAPTER 1

HPV infections and potential outcomes

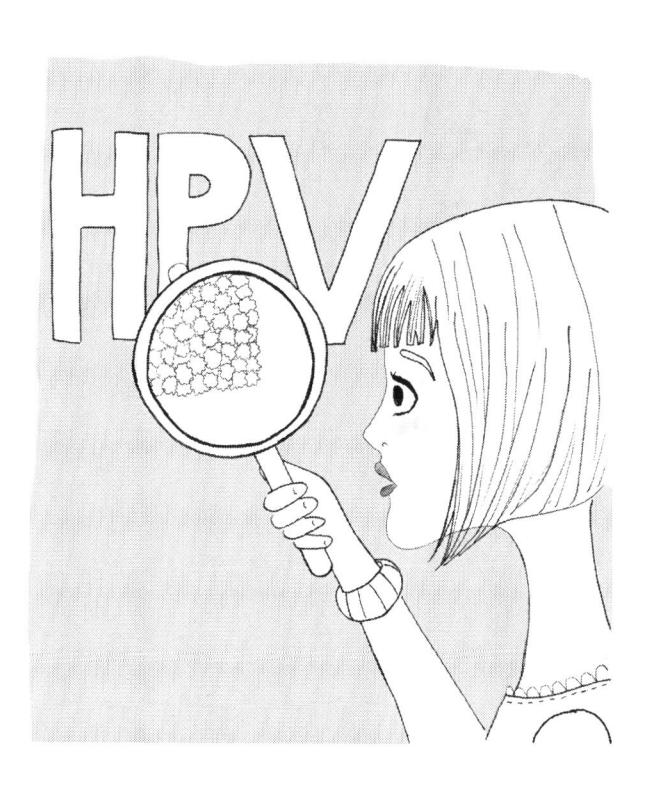

HPV: What it is, where it is and what it causes

1. **What does HPV mean:**
   Human
   Papilloma
   Virus
   HPV is an acronym for the Human Papilloma Virus.

2. **Is it a single virus?**
   No, it is not. More than 100 different types of HPV that infect humans have been identified so far. All differ slightly from each other in their genetic structure.

   HPV types are classified based on the differences in their DNA, i.e. their genetic material (set of genes – genome), into different "genotypes" that are identified by numbers (e.g. HPV 1, 2, 6, 16, etc.). Viruses are the smallest infectious agents, consisting of a genome and its protective shell (protein coating – called capsid). They live and reproduce exclusively in living cells. Figure 1 shows the exterior capsid of HPV and its DNA.

   FIGURE 1: The HPV particle
   The HPV particle has a diameter of 54 nm (1 nm = 1 billionth of one meter) and consists of the DNA, on the inside, and its protective shell (protein coating) or capsid on the outside. The differences in the behavior between HPV types are due to differences in their DNA.

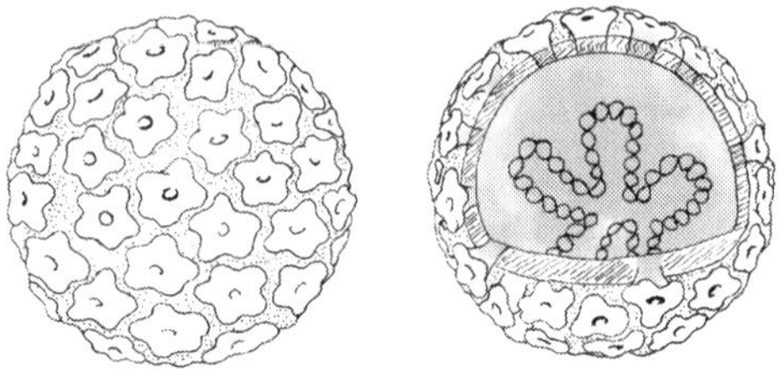

3. What does HPV cause?

It was mentioned above that the different types of HPV are classified based on the differences in their genome (their DNA). These genetic differences dictate their behavior (what area of the body each HPV type prefers to infect and what types of lesions it causes). The term "lesion" means abnormal changes in the structures of tissues due to infection by the HPV.

Most types of HPV infect the skin and cause benign lesions, called warts, on hands, feet, and in other locations. These are called cutaneous HPV types (genotypes 1, 2, 3, 4, 7, 10, etc.)

Another group consists of the genital HPV types (genotypes 6, 11, 16, 18, 31, 33, 45, etc.) which infect the skin lining the lower genital tract, anus, and mouth. Genital HPVs may cause benign lesions, such as warts, as well as precancerous lesions and cancers in the areas they infect.

4. Where do we find HPV?

HPV cannot live in the environment on its own. It can survive on infected materials for just a few hours. HPV lives and multiplies exclusively on humans.

HPV prefers to live and multiply in specific body areas. For example, it can't be found in your blood or in your muscles or bones.

5. On what areas of the human body does HPV live and multiply?

As you know, your body is covered and protected externally by the skin. Mucous membranes have a role similar to the skin and cover wet interior cavities (e.g. mouth, vagina, anus, etc.) (Figure 2).

FIGURE 2: Skin and mucosa
The skin covers the face externally, while the mucous membrane covers the wet cavity of the mouth.

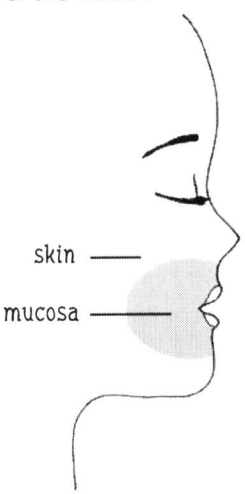

skin ———
mucosa ———

FIGURE 3: Epithelium
The epithelium is the main structural element on the surface of the skin and the mucous membranes. It is the main target of HPV. In Figure 3, we see the squamous epithelium, which is the most common type of epithelium and consists of multiple layers of cells. Epithelial cells sit on a structure called the basement membrane.

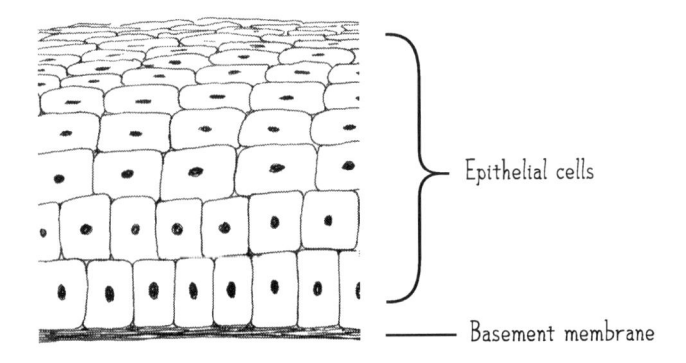

Epithelial cells

Basement membrane

The skin's surface and the mucous membranes are covered by the epithelium (layers of cells with a protective role – called epithelial cells) (Figure 3). Skin is our coat of armor; it protects us from the environment. Mucous membranes have a similar role protecting our internal cavities.

HPV lives and multiplies inside the epithelial cells of the skin and mucous membranes in specific areas of your body.

6. **What are papillomas and what are condylomas?**

Sometimes, infection of the epithelium by certain types of HPV causes hyperplasia (an increase in the number of epithelial cells), creating characteristic growths that protrude from the skin or mucous membranes. Most of these lesions have cauliflower-like projections and are called papillomas (that is where HPV got its name – Human Papilloma Virus -, because it was first identified in papillomas) (Figure 4).

Genital warts are papillomas caused by HPV in the genital area. They are also called condylomas (Latin: condyloma acuminatum, plural: condylomata acuminata).

FIGURE 4: Papilloma (papillae: finger like projection) **with a cauliflower appearance.**

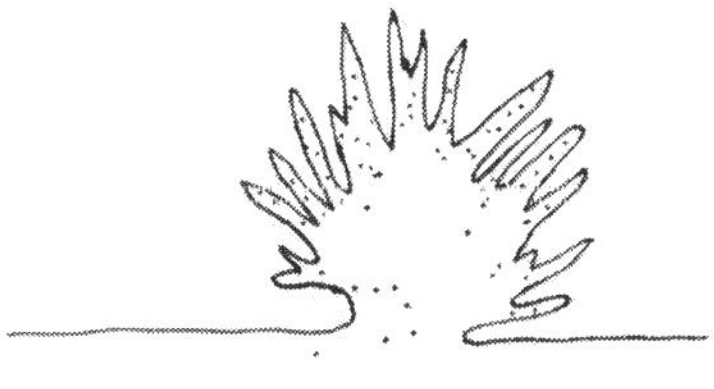

DON'T FORGET:

HPV lives and multiplies only on humans, on the skin and mucous membranes of certain body areas.

It is primarily transmitted through genital skin to genital skin sexual contact.

HPV: Not all types of HPV are the same. Which ones may lead to cancer?

7. **Genital types of HPV: What areas do they infect and what do they cause?**

   A group of different HPV types (approximately 40), referred to as genital types, are of particular interest because it has been proven that they can cause not only papillomas in humans, but also more serious diseases, like precancerous lesions and cancer of various organs.

   Genital types of HPV are transmitted mainly through sexual intercourse. All genital types of HPV, as a group, infect more frequently the epithelium of:
   - the lower genital tract
   - the perianal area and,
   - in rarer cases, the mouth, pharynx, and larynx (figure 5).

   From this point onward, when we refer to HPV we will mean genital types of HPV.

HPV INFECTIONS AND POTENTIAL OUTCOMES 53

FIGURE 5: In what parts of the body do genital types of HPV cause infectious lesions?

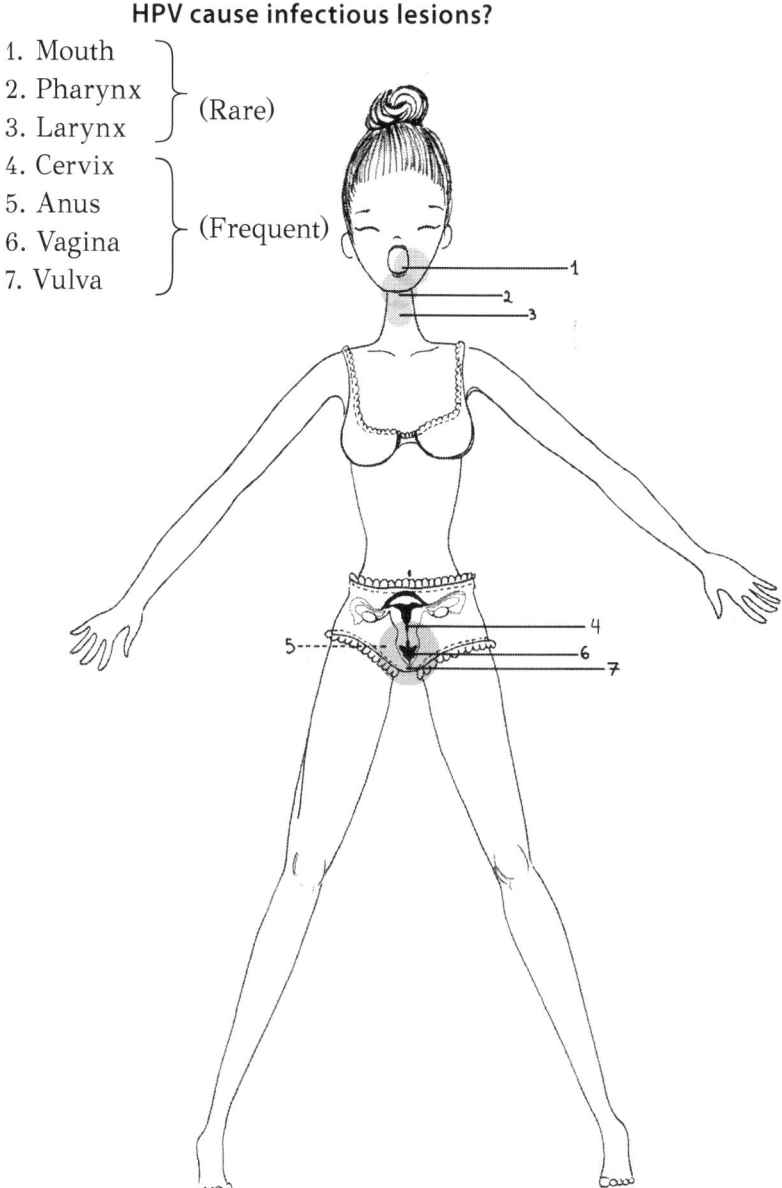

1. Mouth ⎫
2. Pharynx ⎬ (Rare)
3. Larynx ⎭
4. Cervix ⎫
5. Anus   ⎬ (Frequent)
6. Vagina ⎪
7. Vulva   ⎭

8. **Genital types of HPV: Is the specific type important? Are all of them dangerous?**
   Genital types of HPV can be divided into two broad groups: High-risk HPVs and low-risk HPVs, depending upon their association (or lack of association) with cancers. Types that are associated with cancer (high-risk HPVs) are also called oncogenic or HPVs causing cancer. The HPV types not associated with cancer (low-risk HPVs) are called non-oncogenic or non-carcinogenic HPV types.

9. **Low-risk types of HPV: what do they cause?**
   Low-risk types of HPV (6, 11, 42, 43, 44, 54, 61, 70, 72, 81 etc.) cause, as a rule, only benign warty lesions. The most common such lesions are genital warts, also called condylomas (90% of condylomas are caused by HPV 6 and HPV 11).

   HPV 6 and 11 in a few cases cause papillomas in the mouth cavity. They also, very rarely, cause papillomas in the larynx (voice box) and the upper respiratory tract.

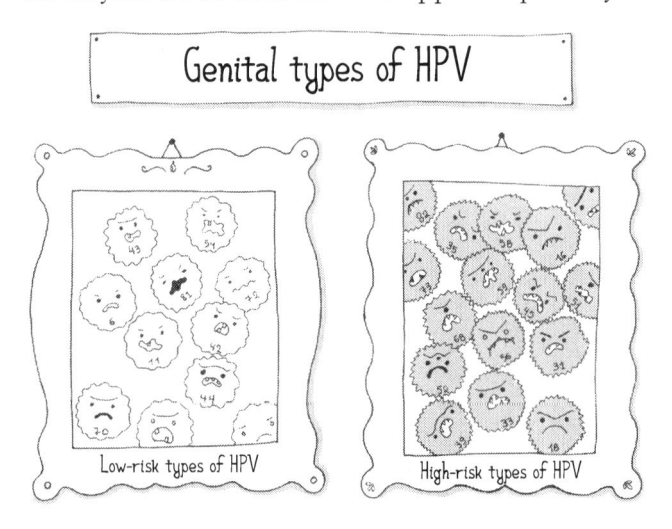

   Genital types of HPV

   Low-risk types of HPV | High-risk types of HPV

Low-risk HPVs may rarely cause recurrent respiratory papillomatosis. Recurrent respiratory papillomatosis (papillomas in the respiratory tract, returning after treatment) is a refractory life-threatening disease but, thankfully, is very rare. Mostly newborns are at risk if they are infected during birth by their mother.

DON'T FORGET:

There is a group of approximately 40 types of HPV, called genital HPV types, which usually infect areas of the genital organs and anus, and, less frequently, the mouth and throat. Genital types of HPV are considered causal factors of warty lesions and cancers.

10. High-risk types of HPV: what do they cause?

High-risk types of HPV (16, 18, 31, 33, 35, 39, 45, 51, 52, 56, 58, 59, 68, 73, 82 etc.), in addition to warty lesions, may also cause precancerous lesions and cancer in various organs (cervix, vagina, vulva, anus, penis, the mouth cavity, tongue, tonsils, pharynx, larynx).

TABLE 1
Genital types of HPV What they can cause

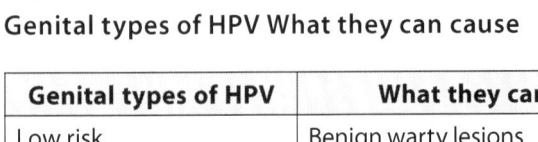

Genital types of HPV	What they can cause
Low risk (6, 11, 42, 43, 44, 54, 61, 70, 72, 81 etc)	Benign warty lesions
High risk (16, 18, 31, 33, 35, 39, 45, 51, 52, 56, 58, 59, 68, 73, 82 etc)	Warty lesions, precancerous lesions and cancer

What can happen to you after the infection?

What happens depends primarily on two factors: the type of the virus and the reaction of your defense system. For most individuals, the immune response appears to dominate and severe lesions never develop. Infected cells may start to grow abnormally as the virus begins to reproduce in large numbers. Whether this occurs at all or not, is largely the result of a complex interplay between the virus and individual immunity.

Short-term: Nothing life-threatening happens.

In a few cases, visible warts will appear, usually within 8 months, if there has been an infection by HPV types that cause genital warts.

In the majority of cases infected generally by genital HPVs, lesions, that are not visible to the naked eye, appear on the epithelium, and cause no symptoms. Most people don't know they are infected because they have only microscopic lesions. These are called subclinical lesions because they cannot be seen by your doctor (during a clinical examination). Most of these lesions are automatically cured by your body and disappear within 2 or 3 years.

Long-term: If you have been infected by an oncogenic type of HPV, there is a risk of carcinogenesis in the coming years (appearance of precancerous lesions or cancer).

11. How does HPV multiply in your cells?

HPV is a parasite of the human body. It takes advantage of the normal cell renewal process in order to multiply (Figures 6a and 6b, pp. 58, 59)

Do you know that you get a new epithelium on your skin approximately every 30 days? The epithelium of the skin and mucous membranes is constantly renewed.

How is it renewed? The surface layer falls off and it is replaced by the cells of the lower layers (Figure 6a).

FIGURE 6A: How the cells multiply and the epithelium is renewed

The cells of the basal layer of the epithelium are divided and new cells are thus produced. As the new cells mature, they move toward the surface of the epithelium. When they finally reach the surface, they have aged, so they die and fall off. The life of each cell is approximately 30 days. And this is how the epithelium is renewed. From the moment you are infected, HPV resides in the cells of the basal layer of the epithelium. As the epithelial cells divide, so does the virus's DNA divide and multiply. If your immune system allows it, it continues to multiply and cause lesions.

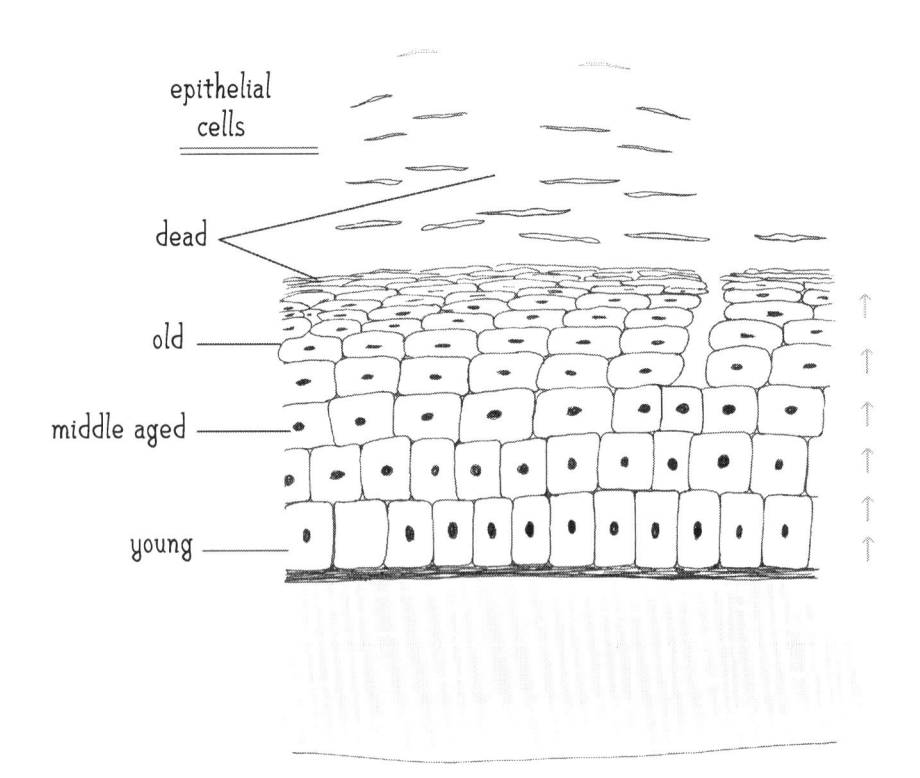

epithelial cells

dead

old

middle aged

young

FIGURE 6B: How does HPV enter the epithelium and start multiplying?

HPV is primarily transmitted through genital skin-to-genital skin sexual contact. HPV infects the epithelium, gaining access to tiny breaks in the skin that often occur during skin-to-skin contact or intercourse. HPV infects the basal layer cells and resides inside the nucleus of the cells. The daughter cells created from the division of the basal layer cells have inside them the HPV DNA. The virus continues to multiply inside the cells, as they mature and move from layer to layer, toward the surface of the epithelium. Until the basal layer cells reach the surface, within the 30 days of their lifetime, thousands of new HPVs have been produced and are released by the dead cells that are on the surface of the epithelium.

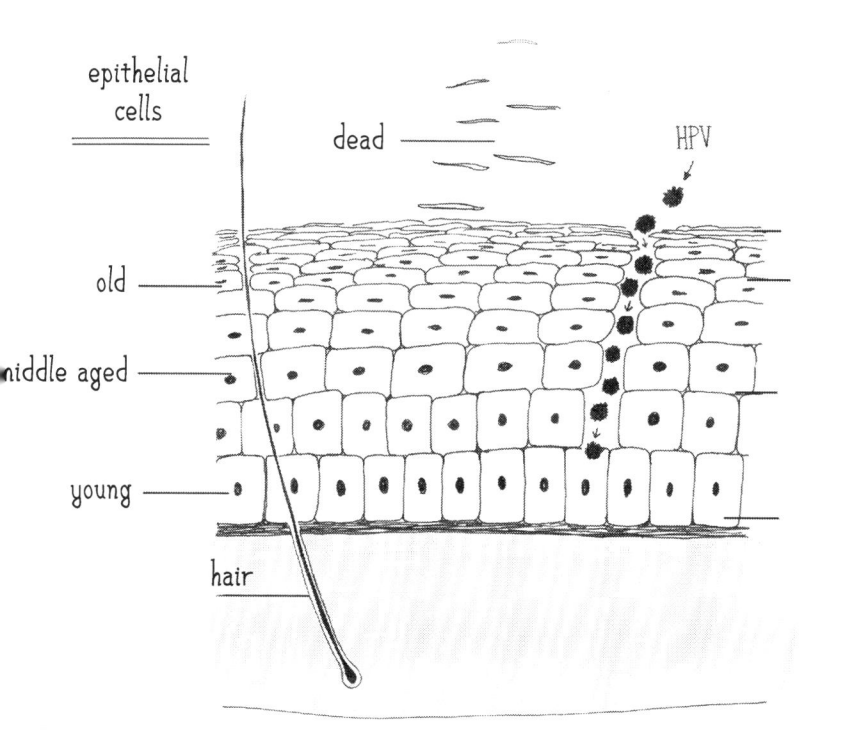

12. If infected, is a lesion certain to occur?

In some women, nothing will happen, and they won't even know they've been infected. Certain people may have an immune system that is strong enough to prevent HPV from multiplying uncontrollably and causing lesions. In these cases, as the basal layer cells multiply into daughter cells, the virus DNA also replicates in small numbers (perhaps 1 HPV per infected cell). Due to its small quantity there is no active infection (lesions) and the virus DNA is undetectable. Such an infection is not traceable with a microscope or an HPV test. This is described as a latent infection (dormant infection). Individuals with latent infection are not considered contagious.

In the majority of infected women though, there is an active viral expression, and the HPV-infected cells begin to change. These cells divide and multiply, creating more HPV-infected cells.

These changes will either manifest as a clinically obvious disease, such as warts, or show as subclinical lesions (lesions not visible to the naked eye). Subclinical lesions are much more common than visible warts. If your immune system allows it, the infectious lesions spread to the entire lower genital tract (vulva, vagina, and cervix).

We don't know why HPV acts more aggressively in some women than in others. Incubation periods (time between exposure to HPV and the appearance of the first lesion) can last from two weeks to eight months or more, with an average of three months.

13. What kinds of lesions may appear in the near future, following the infection?

Depending on the HPV type you are infected with, and the condition of your immune system, one or more of the following may occur:

Invisible lesions (subclinical) on the skin and mucous membranes

This is the most frequent scenario. Invisible infectious lesions appear in the majority of infected individuals. The physician cannot spot them even during a clinical examination, which is why these lesions are called subclinical (they are not visible during a clinical examination). They can be found only with magnifying instruments, like the colposcope or microscope. Usually a biopsy confirms the diagnosis. Another way to identify a subclinical infection is to test directly for the virus' DNA (e.g. with an HPV test taken from the cervix). All genital types of HPV (low- and high-risk) cause subclinical lesions.

Warts (Condylomas or Condylomata acuminata)

In a small percentage (1-3% of HPV infections in general), HPV infection (mostly by HPVs 6 and 11) results, in addition to subclinical lesions, in the simultaneous appearance of genital warts. Warts protrude from the skin and the mucous membranes, and vary in size. They are usually visible to the naked eye. Many of them are "cauliflower" shaped. Visible warts are also called condylomata acuminata. They are caused by HPV6 and HPV11 in 90% of the cases.

Both subclinical lesions and warts have the same "microscopic characteristics" when looking at the structure of cells through the microscope, and are described by the terms condylomatous (warty) HPV lesions or with the international term LSIL (Low-grade Squamous Intraepithelial lesion) (see question 27 p. 68).

DON'T FORGET:

In summary, two kinds of lesions may appear in HPV-infected individuals, usually within a few months after the infection, and they are:
- subclinical (invisible to the naked eye) lesions (more frequent)
- visible warts (in relatively few cases)

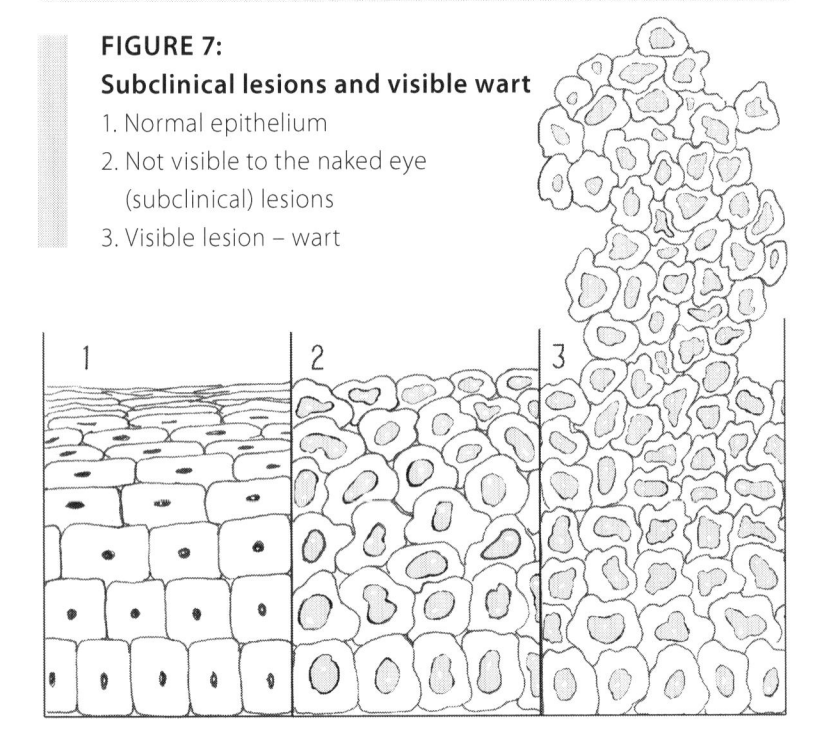

FIGURE 7:
Subclinical lesions and visible wart
1. Normal epithelium
2. Not visible to the naked eye (subclinical) lesions
3. Visible lesion – wart

14. If you are infected today, when will the first lesions appear?

They usually appear within the first 6 months after the infection. This is what studies of visible genital wart cases have shown. There are, however, a few cases where warty lesions appear much later. The immune system obviously initially suppressed the virus (in latent form – latent infection), but when it later weakened, the infection on the epithelium flared up and lesions started appearing.

15. What happens after genital warts appear?

The first wart usually appears within a few weeks or several months after the day you were infected.

Your immune system tries to suppress the infection. Until it manages to do so (which may take over 12 months), it is likely you will see new warts appearing. In a small percentage of patients it has been observed that warts subside spontaneously within a one-year period.

16. Are genital warts life-threatening?

No, they are not life-threatening under any circumstance. Genital warts, as a rule, are benign.

17. If you have invisible (subclinical) lesions from HPV on the cervix at this time, how can you know about it?

You cannot know it. They are not visible and do not cause any symptoms.

The only way to find these lesions is to have a Pap test, an HPV test, a colposcopy or a biopsy. If you have regular check-ups and you find that you have an IIPV infection, your physician will advise you about what tests you must have after that.

Most people infected with HPV are not aware of it because they have no symptoms and the subclinical lesions on the skin and mucous membranes are not visible.

18. **Are you at direct risk from the invisible lesions caused immediately after the infection?**

    No, you are not at risk immediately after the infection. Subclinical lesions are usually suppressed by your body spontaneously. They have been studied at length on the uterine cervix and it has been proven that:
    - In women infected with HPV, the active infection subsided spontaneously in 80-90% of cases within 2-3 years.
    - Only in cases with persistent and recurring infection from oncogenic types of HPV is there a risk for developing cancer.

How and when will HPV infection lead to cancer?

19. **How can HPV drive your cells crazy?**

    After the persistent infection of your cells by one or more high-risk types of HPV, the virus DNA can be incorporated into the DNA of certain cells. This essentially means that mutated cells are created in your body.

Of course, your body can repair or destroy a few mutated cells. There are special tumor-suppressor mechanisms, but they are not always successful.

The problem with high-risk types of HPV is that they not only cause mutations, but also neutralize the tumor-suppressor mechanisms we all have. In a next stage, if there are multiple mutations, your body loses control completely. The mutated cells multiply autonomously and uncontrollably at a fast pace and create tumors.

INFECTIONS AND CANCER:

A significant percentage of cancers in humans (18-20%) are the result of chronic infections that are caused by viruses, bacteria, and parasites.
Such examples are liver cancer in cases of chronic infection from the hepatitis virus, stomach cancer from helicobacter pylori, Kaposi sarcoma and non-Hodgkin's lymphoma in cases of AIDS, lymphomas related to HIV and Epstein-Barr virus etc. It has been calculated that HPVs are responsible for 5% of cancer cases in humans.

20. What is the most frequent cancer in women caused by HPV?

Cervical cancer is the most frequent cancer caused by HPV. It is estimated that there are 500,000 new cervical cancer cases each year, worldwide. Half of these women lose their life. This is considered a major health problem, since this cancer usually appears in young women.

21. Which women are at a higher risk for cervical cancer?

The cervix is the organ that has been studied at great length with regard to carcinogenesis caused by HPV. Among women infected with oncogenic HPV, 10% do not manage to easily suppress the infection or prevent recurrences.

This small percentage of women is at a higher risk of developing premalignant lesions and cervical cancer in the future.

Therefore, it has been documented that persistent and recurring infections of the cervix by oncogenic types of HPV may cause cancer (carcinogenesis).

22. If a woman is infected with an oncogenic type of HPV, will cervical cancer develop immediately?

No. Carcinogenesis in the cervix is a drawn-out process. Several years intervene between the infection and the appearance of cancer.

23. Why is cervical cancer considered preventable?

- Because premalignant lesions usually appear before cancer does, and they can be found and treated.

- If women have regular check-ups with Pap smears and HPV tests, those premalignant lesions are found.

- Mass screening using Pap tests in the Western world has reduced cervical cancer incidence by 80-90%.

- Pap tests discover suspicious cells. The HPV test finds out whether there is an infection from oncogenic types of HPV in the cervix. If the check-up (screening tests such as Pap test and HPV test) comes up with any findings, women then undergo an examination called a colposcopy. Premalignant lesions are identified and treated.

- It is believed that the combination of preventive vaccination for HPV, together with routine screening, will minimize future risk in young girls.

24. How can a woman know that she is not at risk?

If she is having regular check-ups and there are no suspicious findings then she is not at risk. If there are premalignant lesions, they will be discovered with the Pap test, the HPV test, and the colposcopy and they will be treated.

25. In what organs, other than the cervix, can high-risk types of HPV cause cancer?

In women, genital high-risk types of HPV (oncogenic types of HPV), beside cervical cancer, can cause cancer of the vulva, vagina, anus and head and neck. Cancers that are known collectively as head and neck cancers usually begin in the squamous cells that line the moist, mucosal surfaces inside the head and neck (for example inside the mouth, the throat, the base of the tongue and the tonsils).

In men, HPV can cause cancer of the penis, anus, and head and neck.

These cancers are rarer than cervical cancer. There is a detailed reference to the cancers caused by HPV in various organs in chapter 10.

26. How can doctors tell the difference between premalignant lesions and simple infections?

Accurate diagnosis always requires tissue examination through the microscope.

The entire thickness of the epithelium must be examined to get an accurate diagnosis. This is why, if there is any suspicion, biopsies are performed (see Figure 12, p. 129).

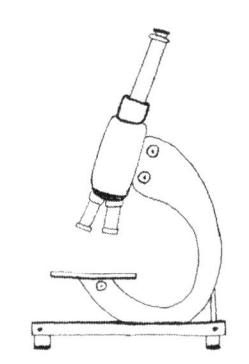

In simple infections, the epithelium does not lose its normal structure. The epithelial layers are in order, and the cells change as they mature and move from the basal layer to the surface.

In premalignant lesions, the epithelium loses its normal structure and two-thirds or its whole thickness is occupied by cells with atypical nuclei (see figures a-h in pages 160, 161)

27. What are LSIL and HSIL?

Lesions caused by HPVs, with the characteristics of benign infection, are internationally called LSIL (from the initials of the words Low-grade Squamous Intraepithelial Lesions).

Precancerous lesions caused by HPVs are internationally called HSIL (High-grade Squamous Intraepithelial Lesions).

Genital types of HPV: How are they transmitted?

28. Where is the HPV that will infect you located?

As already mentioned, HPV lives and multiplies only on humans. On an infected person, HPV is found on the surface of infected epithelia (usually in the genital organs and perianal area).

The epithelia most commonly infected are those that sustain more friction during sexual contact.

29. How are genital types of HPV transmitted?

HPV is primarily transmitted from one person to another through genital skin – to genital skin sexual contact.

Vaginal or anal intercourse are the main ways of transmission (Table 2, p. 70).

However, any type of friction with an individual's infected skin or mucous membranes can lead to transmission of the virus to another person. It is not necessary to have penetration during sexual intercourse to transmit the virus.

HPV can also be transmitted through oral-genital contact, friction with infected fingers (mutual masturbation) or shared use of sex toys.

There is no evidence that contaminated toilet seats, doorknobs, towels, soaps, swimming pools or hot tubs can transmit genital HPVs. However, some unexplained cases of HPV lesions do occur and one should never rule out the possibility that an HPV infection may have been transmitted in a non-sexual event.

The infection usually spreads to neighboring areas, e.g. from the vulva to the vagina and the cervix. The infection that initially appeared in the genitals may later spread to the anal area.

It is possible to transfer the infection from one area to another with infected fingers. This usually happens by scratching the infected area and then a neighboring area. This spreading of the infection from one area to another by the fingers (on the same person) is called auto-inoculation.

TABLE 2
Ways of transmitting the infection with genital types of HPV

It is highly possible to become infected through:	Vaginal intercourse without condom Anal intercourse without condom
You have a relatively smaller chance of becoming infected with HPV through:	Vaginal or anal intercourse with condom Oral-genital contact Friction of the genital area with genitals (without penetration), infected objects (sex toys) or fingers
You have a very small chance of becoming infected with HPV through:	Shared use of dirty towels or underwear with infected individuals
You will not contract HPV:	From a toilet seat From door-knobs, handles, faucets, etc.

In relatively rare cases, the virus can be transmitted from the pregnant mother to the newborn during birth. Most clinicians believe that the risk of cesarean section to both mother and baby exceeds the risk of the baby acquiring respiratory papillomatosis (HPV 6 or 11 induced warts in the larynx or upper airway – see page 153). Once warts are no longer present, especially if a woman has had no detectable HPV lesions for 6 months or more, transmission of HPV to the baby during vaginal delivery becomes increasingly unlikely.

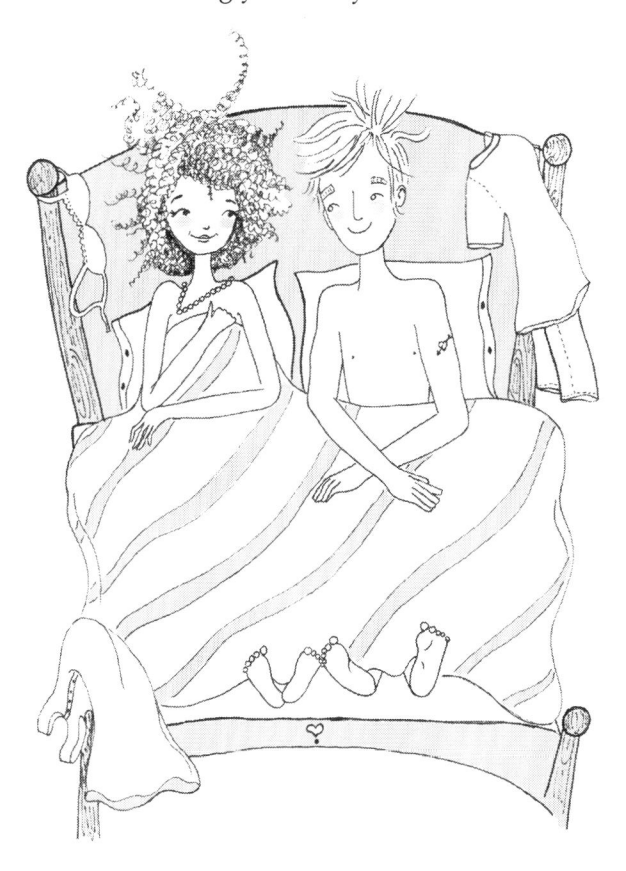

WHEN WILL THE VIRUS NOT INFECT YOU?

If you have been vaccinated, the antibodies you have developed for the HPV types that are covered by your vaccine won't allow these viruses to enter your cells and cause infection.

Oncogenic types of HPV: Sneaky invaders – Dangerous roommates. What can you do?

30. **Can you know if you have been infected in the past by an oncogenic type of HPV or if you have an active infection in your cervical cells right now?**
    Not always. If the HPV test in a woman shows that there is an infection by oncogenic types of HPV in the cervix, the diagnosis is certain. There is no way, however, to know when the infection started.

    We know that women who had premalignant lesions in the past have certainly been infected by oncogenic types of HPV.

31. **If an HPV infection is suppressed, does the risk continue to exist?**
    If the infection was caused by oncogenic HPV types, there is sometimes a risk of recurrence of the infection and carcinogenesis.

32. Does HPV ever leave your body? Do you have to keep having check-ups?

Studies show that, in most women who were infected in the cervix, the HPV DNA cannot be detected after 2 or 3 years.

There are, however, cases where the virus is reactivated, many years later, and causes infection again. The virus has obviously remained inside cells all those years.

We cannot know in which cases this may occur. This is why all women must have regular check-ups.

33. How can HPV appear again after many years?

It is believed that, after suppression of the lesions, the virus DNA remains in small quantities in the cells of the basal layer of the epithelium. Some basal cells may actually serve as a long-lived reservoir of HPV infection (see Figure 6b, page 59).

As we said above, this is called a latent infection. In latent infection cases, the HPV DNA cannot be detected with the tests we have available. If your immune system allows it, the virus can become active again and cause infection once more. This means that the risk for carcinogenesis recurs.

34. Once with HPV – always with HPV?

Most of the information we have suggests that the HPV test (which detects HPV infection) become negative over time in most women.

Whether an immune-mediated regression clears the HPV from the body completely or just suppresses it to the point where it is not likely to be contagious nor cause HPV-induced disease in the future is not known for sure.

So, if you were once infected by the HPV virus, its reactivation cannot be ruled out. HPV may be dormant in your body for several years and then reactivate if your body's immunity is compromised. Therefore, routine check-ups are necessary for every woman.

35. How do you explain that many people are infected by HPV viruses but only a few have serious problems from them?

The type of the virus plays an important role. However, the immune system (the human body's defense mechanism) and the good function of the body's tumor-suppressing mechanisms are more important.

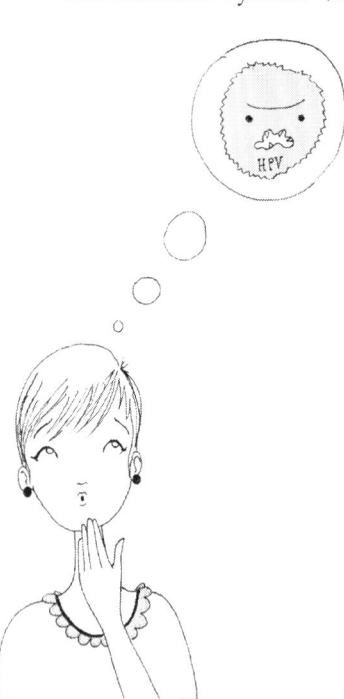

For example, HPV 16 is the most oncogenic type of HPV and causes persistent infections. We know, however, that many women infected with HPV 16 on the cervix suppress the infection within 2-3 years without any consequences. Despite this, in some cases infections from HPV 16 on the cervix are persistent. It is obvious that the immune system of these women cannot control and suppress them. A significant percentage of these women will develop premalignant lesions and, later on, cervical cancer.

We cannot know what exactly the body's reaction to an HPV infection will be or which individuals are more sensitive than others. The only thing that can be done is implement prevention policies.

36. How can a woman know that she is not at risk?
If the testing for active infection from oncogenic types of HPV is negative (HPV test), it is likely that she is not at risk in the immediate future.

However, there is always a risk of an old infection flaring up again or of a new infection by some other type of HPV which she is not aware of. Therefore, in order to protect her health she must undergo routine check-ups (HPV test and/or Pap test).

What are your chances of becoming infected by genital types of HPV?

37. How frequent are HPV infections in the population?
HPV infections are very frequent. They are the most frequent sexually transmitted infections.

Many estimates have placed the lifetime likelihood of getting genital HPV to be in the range of 75-90%.

The highest rates of active infection on the cervix by one or more types of HPV are found in young women aged 18-25 years old and range between 25% and 35%. This is explained by the frequent change of sexual partners.

The risk of exposure to HPV is estimated to be approximately 12-25% per partner.

The rates of active infections drop significantly as the age increases (5-10% in women 40-50 years old).

In the majority of cases with HPV infections there are only subclinical lesions that cannot be seen with the "naked" eye.

Approximately 1-3% of the population has genital warts, and the lifetime risk is estimated to be about 10%.

38. Does the chance of infection by genital types of HPV increase depending on the number of sexual partners?

American researchers studied a large group of female students for at least five years. The study included female students who started having sexual contact within the 6 months prior to being included in the study and it focused on infection percentages over time (the uterine cervix was tested for HPV DNA every 6 months). It was found that, within the first two years, 60% of the students were infected by one or more types of HPV, and within five years 80% of them had been infected. The infection percentages were proportional to the reported number of sexual partners.

It is self-evident that the restriction of the number of sexual partners reduces the risk of infection.

39. What is the probability of becoming infected by a new partner?

It is considered that the risk of exposure to HPV is 12-25% for each new sexual partner. To get infected, your partner must have an active infection.

THE MOST COMMON SCENARIO IN MOST OF THE UNFORTUNATE CASES OF CERVICAL CANCER IS THE FOLLOWING:

A young woman was once infected by an oncogenic type of HPV, let's say at around the age of 25. She had no symptoms –which is usually the case– and was therefore unaware of the infection. The virus caused lesions on her cervix. The infectious lesions persisted a long period of time or may have originally subsided and recurred later.

During a phase when the infection was active, the HPV managed to cause mutations in the cells of the epithelium. A premalignant lesion was thus formed. The woman was unaware of it, since premalignant lesions from HPV usually cause no symptoms.

All these years, from the age of 25 to 35, this woman was not consistent with her check-ups. She had no PAP smears (to find any suspicious cells), and, of course, no HPV tests (to detect cancer-causing HPVs).

The premalignant lesions evolved into cancer. The woman sought medical advice when she was 35, because she now had symptoms (blood from the vagina, odorous discharge, blood after intercourse, etc.). Invasive cervical cancer was diagnosed. When these symptoms appear it is usually too late...

40. **Can you know if your partner has an active infection at this time?**

Not usually. Most infectious lesions caused by HPV are invisible and cause no symptoms. Infected individuals are usually not aware of it.

Only genital warts are visible and you can take preventive measures against becoming infected. Visible genital warts are highly infectious (60-70% transmission rate).

41. **Are there high-risk sexual partners?**

Yes, there are. It has been proven that people who report a high number of sexual partners may be hosting one or more types of HPV. Also, people with compromised immune systems (e.g. AIDS patients) have persistent infections from HPV more frequently. Therefore, as regards the risk of infection, the choice of sexual partner plays an important role.

42. **What is the possibility of a person becoming infected by HPV over his or her lifetime?**

The chance of infection by one or more types of HPV depends on the number of sexual partners and on the sexual history of these partners. It is not the same for all individuals. An exact percentage cannot, of course, be cited. Based on the current sexual practices of young people in the western world, the chance of infection up to the age of 50 is estimated to be higher than 90%.

> **DON'T FORGET:**
>
> Limiting the number of sexual partners reduces the risk of infection.
>
> The choice of sexual partner plays an important role.
>
> Use of a condom reduces the risk of infection by up to 70%.

43. Does the use of a condom prevent HPV infection?

The use of a condom does reduce the possibility of an HPV infection (up to 70% according to all publications), but does not completely eliminate it. The reasons are obvious:

- A condom does not cover the entire surface of the penis. There may be lesions in the surrounding areas (testicles, pubis, perineum) where there is contact during intercourse.
- A condom is not used strictly in all sexual contacts or throughout the duration of intercourse.

Even though a condom does not fully protect from the risk of HPV infection, its use is recommended even for the partial protection it offers.

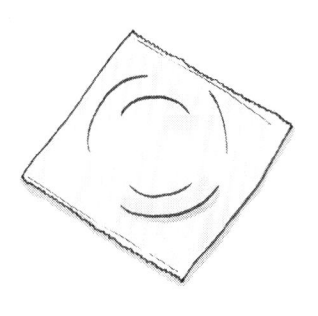

In any event, it protects from other, very serious, sexually transmitted diseases.

What can you do to protect your health?

44. What does prevention entail?
There are two types of prevention, primary and secondary.

45. What is primary prevention?
Primary prevention involves not letting HPV infect you. How can one ensure this?
- a) By vaccination (that protects from specific types of HPV).
- b) By practicing safe sexual behavior (limiting the number of sexual partners, careful choice of sexual partners and use of a condom).

46. What is secondary prevention?
Secondary prevention involves having routine check-ups to prevent, in time, any consequences of an infection and choosing a healthy lifestyle and diet to boost your immune system.

Secondary prevention is being successfully implemented against cervical cancer. Women are preventively tested using Pap tests and HPV tests, which help detect and treat premalignant lesions (Table 3, p. 81).

All the above make clear the value of prevention. Over the next five chapters we will discuss in detail the various prevention methods.

It is interesting to note that, thanks to all the means available today, cervical cancer is nearly 100% preventable, and we can prevent other cancers caused by HPV at rates higher than 90%.

TABLE 3
Prevention of infection by HPV and its complications

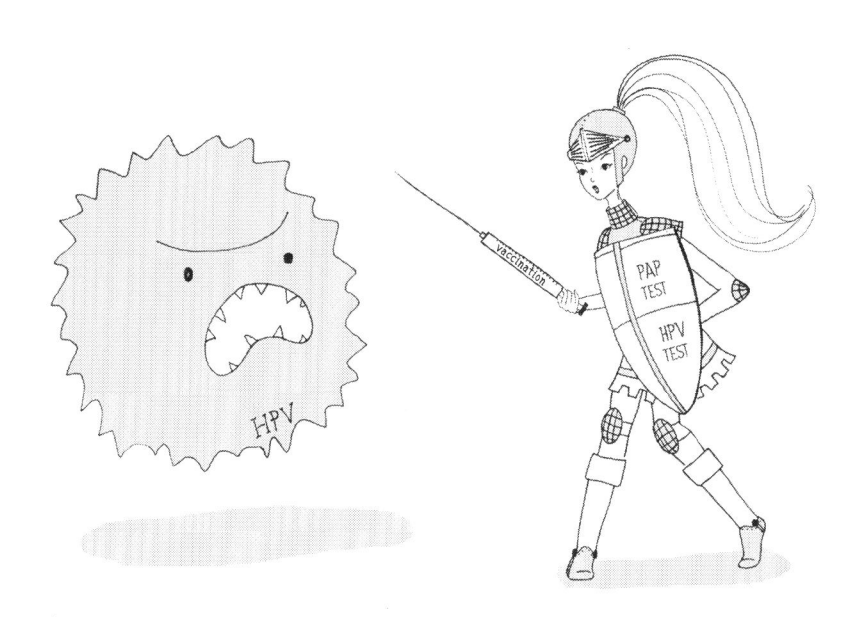

Primary Prevention	Secondary Prevention
(reducing the chances of infection) • Preventive vaccination • Limiting the number of sexual partners • Use of condoms	(mainly implemented for cervical cancer) • Pap test • HPV test • Colposcopy, Biopsy

CHAPTER 2

Prevention of infection from specific types of HPV with vaccination

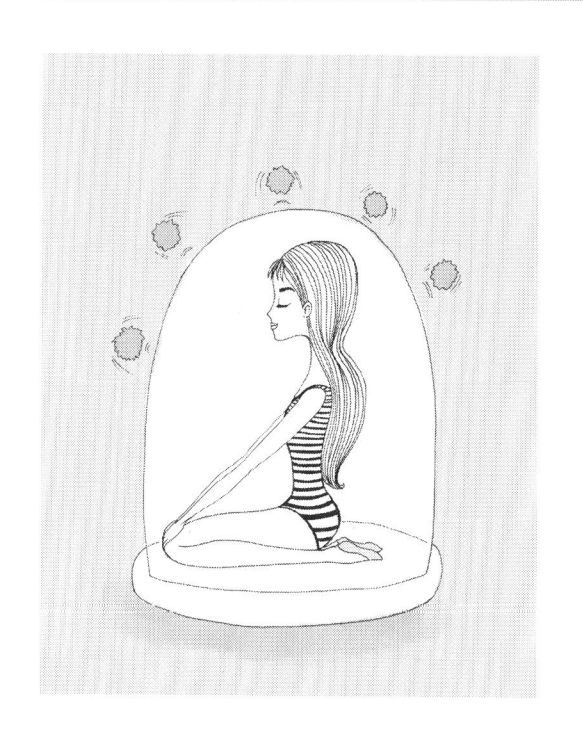

We know that genital warts appear as a result of infection by a certain group of genital types of HPV. We also believe that infection by another group of genital types of HPV (oncogenic types) is causally related to carcinogenesis in the lower reproductive system and the anal area. It has been proven that preventive vaccination for specific types of HPV is highly successful in preventing genital warts as well as precancerous lesions caused by the types for which each vaccine has been designed.

47. Which vaccines have been made available to date?

In 2006, a quadrivalent vaccine (Gardasil) became the first commercially available HPV vaccine, targeting high-risk HPV types 16 and 18, which alone account for 70% of cervical cancers, as well as low-risk HPVs 6 and 11, which are predominantly responsible (90% of cases) for genital warts.

A bivalent vaccine (Cervarix) was released in 2007 in Europe and in 2009 in the United States. It targets high-risk types 16 and 18.

More recently, Gardasil 9 was licensed for use by the Food and Drug Administration (FDA) in the United States (December 2014). This newest vaccine targets the 7 most common cancer-causing subtypes (16, 18, 31, 33, 45, 52, and 58) which account for more than 90% of HPV-related cancers, as well as subtypes 6 and 11 (which account for 90% of case of genital warts).

48. How do vaccines against HPV work?

The vaccines stimulate the immune system to produce antibodies against the HPV genotypes for which they were designed. If an individual is vaccinated before becoming infected and antibodies are produced, then the virus can not cause an infection.

49. Do the vaccines prevent against all types of HPV?
No, they do not cover you against all types of HPV. It would be impossible to create a vaccine that covers 40 different viruses. They were designed and created to protect you against those types of HPV that cause the most problems.

50. Which types of HPV do vaccines protect you from?

Gardasil
The first Gardasil vaccine became available in 2006, and it protects against HPV 6, 11, 16 and 18. The production of this vaccine was based on the prevention of genital warts (which in 90% of the cases are caused by HPV 6 and 11) and the majority of cervical cancers (which in 70% of cases are caused by HPV 16 and 18).

Cervarix
Cervarix became available in 2007 with the goal of protecting against HPV 16 and 18. According to studies published later, it was proven that Cervarix provided partial coverage (due to cross protection) also from types 31, 33, and 45.

Gardasil 9
In December of 2014, the Food and Drug Administration (FDA) in the USA approved the Gardasil 9 vaccine. Gardasil 9 covers against types 6, 11, 16, 18, 31, 33, 45, 52, and 58, offering clearly greater coverage compared to the previous vaccines.

WANTED

HPV 6 HPV 11
Responsible for 90% of genital warts

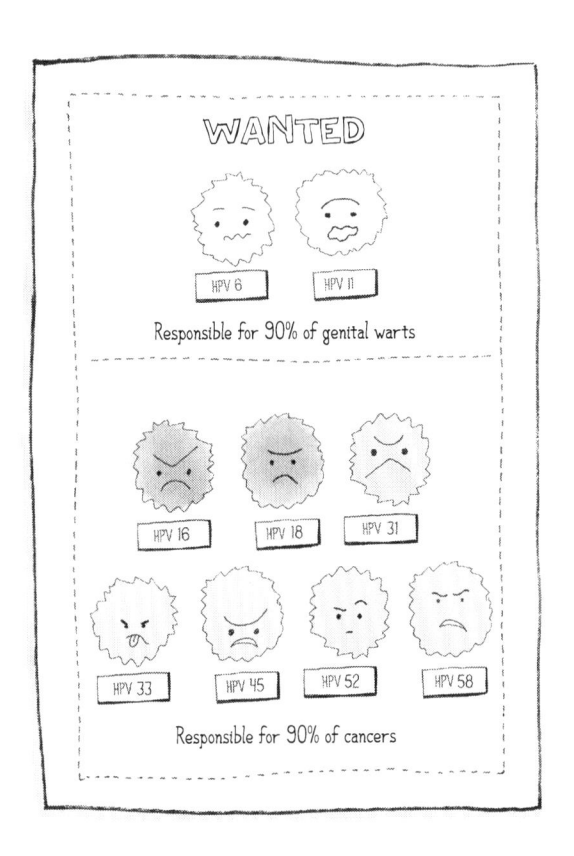

HPV 16 HPV 18 HPV 31
HPV 33 HPV 45 HPV 52 HPV 58
Responsible for 90% of cancers

51. Which HPV-related diseases do the vaccines protect you from?

Genital warts

In 90% of genital wart cases, low-risk HPV types 6 and 11 are detected, while other types of HPV are detected in the remaining 10% (also oncogenic ones). Gardasil has been proven to provide a 92% protection against genital warts.

Cervical cancer

It is estimated that in all cervical cancer cases attributed to HPV:
- 70% of cases are caused by HPV 16 and 18 and
- 20% of cases are caused by HPV 31, 33, 45, 52, and 58.
- The other oncogenic types of HPV are responsible for the remaining 10%.

According to these data, the first Gardasil vaccine covers 70% of cervical cancer cases, while the new Gardasil 9 protects against 90% of cervical cancer cases, because it protects from infection with HPV 16, 18, 31, 33, 45, 52, and 58.

Other cancers

It is calculated that the seven oncogenic types of HPV (16, 18, 31, 33, 45, 52, and 58) which are covered by Gardasil 9, are also responsible for:
- 95% of anal cancers and
- 85% of vaginal and vulvar cancers (among cancers attributed to HPV).

It is anticipated that there will be a similar decrease in the probability of the above diseases in children who will be vaccinated with Gardasil 9.

52. How was the effectiveness of the vaccines proven?

We know that carcinogenesis from genital types of HPV in the lower reproductive system and the anus is a drawn out process, and that premalignant lesions appear before invasive cancer does.

The studies conducted before the first vaccines became available proved their effectiveness in preventing premalignant lesions that lead to cervical cancer (as well as genital warts in the case of Gardasil).

The studies on Gardasil 9 focused from the start on the prevention of premalignant lesions in multiple organs:
- in women (uterine cervix, vagina, vulva, and anus)
- and in men (anus and penis)

as well as on the prevention of genital warts in women and men.

The vaccine was proven 100% effective as regards the prevention of the above lesions caused by the 9 types of HPV it protects from.

53. What about head and neck cancers attributed to HPV?

It is believed that oncogenic types of HPV (mainly HPV 16) are the causal factors in 25-35% of head and neck cancers (mouth cavity, base of tongue, tonsils, pharynx, and larynx). We are not fully aware, however, of the exact carcinogenesis process in this area as compared to the cervix (premalignant lesions which develop into cancer if left untreated). Therefore, the vaccine cannot officially be recommended, since there are no studies on the prevention of head and neck cancers.

Head and neck cancers usually appear after the age of 50. The beneficial coverage of the vaccine is therefore expected to be proven at a later date, if the incidence of these cancers drops in people who were vaccinated when they were children and teenagers.

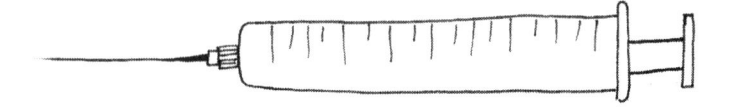

54. Do the vaccines contain viruses?

The vaccines contain no HPV DNA. They contain virus like particles made from proteins manufactured in the laboratory to simulate the external capsid of HPV. These Virus-Like Particles (VLPs) stimulate your immune system to produce antibodies. In reality they "trick" the human body, which perceives the VLPs as real HPV and starts producing antibodies. It has been proven that antibodies created by this process do not allow the real HPV to cause infection, with all the possible consequences.

55. Are vaccines a method of prevention or a method of treatment?

Vaccines are a method of prevention. As mentioned above they provide protection against specific types of HPV, on condition that you were not infected in the past by those specific HPV types.

56. Should boys be vaccinated?

Yes, they should. The vaccination of boys will protect them from genital warts and most cancers caused by HPV in men.

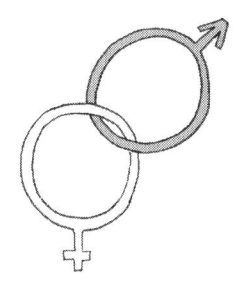

It is believed that the simultaneous vaccination of boys and girls will greatly reduce the frequency of infections and, in the future, of cancers caused by oncogenic types of HPV.

57. What is the ideal age for vaccination?
The recommendation is that boys and girls are vaccinated between the ages of 11-26. It is believed that the best prevention is achieved when all children are vaccinated (boys and girls) between the ages of 11-12. Vaccination at this age has the following advantages:
- Sexual activity has not started yet. If the 3 doses of the vaccine are administered before the start of any sexual activity, the benefits are greater. According to two studies in the USA, a significant number of girls have started their sexual activity at the age of 12. In a study in Sweden, it was proven that the efficacy of vaccination in preventing genital warts was 93% in the group of girls vaccinated between 10-13 years old. In the group vaccinated at the age of 20-22, it was 48% and, finally, at the 23-26-year-old group it was 21%.
- It has been proven that immunization (production of antibodies against the HPV viruses) is more effective at these young ages. Antibody levels after vaccination were compared in two groups of girls and young women. The first group included girls aged 9-14 years old and the second young women 15-26 years old. In the first group, the antibody levels were clearly higher than those of the second group.

58. Is vaccination recommended even after the beginning of sexual activity?

If a teenager has already started engaging in sexual activity, this does not mean that he or she has been infected by all the types of HPV covered by the vaccine. Therefore, vaccination in older ages is recommended, to prevent any new infections.

59. How is the vaccine administered? Trends and most recent estimates

It is administered in 3 doses (injected intramuscularly), within a 6-month period.

In the USA medical organizations (FDA, CDC, ACIP) recommend a two-dose regimen of the HPV vaccine Gardasil-9 for boys and girls aged 9 to 14 years old.

The FDA approval was based on results of a clinical trial funded by Merck, which manufactures Gardasil 9. The trial showed that a two-dose regimen of the vaccine in 9- to 14-year-olds produced an antibody response similar to or greater than that produced by a three-dose regimen in 16- to 26-year-old women.

Merck is no longer marketing its older quadrivalent Gardasil vaccine, which protects against infection by four HPV types, in the United States. And GlaxoSmithKline, which manufactures Cervarix, an HPV vaccine that protects against two high-risk HPV types, announced in October 2016 that it will no longer sell its vaccine.

60. **How safe are the vaccines?**
    We have enough data available to confirm the safety of vaccines. The first vaccine (Gardasil) became available in 2006, and Cervarix in 2007. It is a known fact that vaccines are tested for many years before they reach the market. Scientific data available today on the safety of vaccines are based not only on the trial phase, but also the reporting of their side effects after they are made available to the public and after many millions of doses are administered.
    According to announcements by internationally recognized health organizations regarding the control of vaccines (like the FDA), no serious side effects connected with the use of the vaccines were observed in vaccinated women in the USA (2006-2016, 70 million doses).
    Based on the above data, vaccines are considered to have a safe profile.
    Like all vaccines, even "old" vaccines approved many years ago, the HPV vaccines are continuously monitored for side effects. The US Centers for Disease Control and Prevention (CDC) and the US Food and Drug Administration (FDA) review all serious side effects reported to the Vaccine Adverse Event Reporting System (VAERS) to watch for potential safety concerns that may need further study.

61. **What are the side effects of the vaccines?**
    As mentioned above, from our experience to date, HPV vaccines are considered well-tolerated and safe. The following side effects have been reported in order of frequency:

- Local reaction at the point of injection (pain, redness, and swelling).
- Fever (usually mild), headache.
- Feeling faint immediately after the injection. It is known that fainting episodes may occur after any type of injection. Faintness was observed more frequently in teenage girls, after their vaccination. To avoid any injury from fainting it is recommended that the girl remains lying on her back for 15 minutes after the injection.
- Muscle pain, fatigue, gastrointestinal disorders, and other mild side effects have been reported much more rarely.
- Allergic-type reactions. On very rare occasions, severe (anaphylactic) allergic reactions may occur after vaccination. People with severe allergies to any component of a vaccine should not receive that vaccine.
- There have been reported rare cases of ovarian dysfunction after receiving Gardasil vaccine. This is under investigation.

62. Indications for the new Gardasil 9

Gardasil 9 is recommended for girls and women aged 9-26 to prevent the following diseases:
- Cancer of the uterine cervix, vagina, vulva, and anus caused by HPVs 16, 18, 31, 33, 45, 52, and 58.
- Premalignant lesions in the above organs (CIN, AIS, VaIN, VIN, AIN) from the specific types of HPV.
- Genital warts caused by HPV 6 and 11.

Gardasil 9 is also recommended for boys 9-15 years old to prevent the following diseases:

- Anal cancer and premalignant lesions (AIN) caused by HPV 16, 18, 31, 33, 45, 52 and 58.
- Genital warts caused by HPV 6 and 11.

63. **What do we know about the vaccine during pregnancy?**
There are no studies on the safety of the vaccine in pregnant women. From isolated cases, it appears that there is no risk to the pregnant woman or the fetus. However, vaccination is not recommended during pregnancy.

64. **What happens if a woman becomes pregnant before completing the three doses?**
It is recommended that the other doses are administered after the end of the pregnancy. There is no contraindication for the mother or the baby during breastfeeding.

65. **After they are vaccinated, should women continue to have check-ups?**
Women who were vaccinated must continue to have regular check-ups (screening with Pap test and/or HPV test). Women should be informed that no vaccine can provide 100% coverage since it does not protect against all oncogenic types of HPV.

66. **Is there a therapeutic vaccine for HPV?**
Efforts are made to produce therapeutic vaccines but there is no such possibility yet.

67. **Do vaccines lead to increased sexual activity in young people?**
Concerns around HPV vaccination have been expressed and published in academic journals and other media. The

hypothesis was expressed that HPV vaccination will create a false sense of protection from sexually transmitted diseases in young people, which will result in an increase in their sexual activity, starting earlier and not using protection.

Published studies have shown that there is no evidence to support such concerns.

68. Is an HPV DNA test recommended before the vaccination?

No, it is not. This question is frequently asked by girls and women with an active sexual life. It is reasonable that they want to know if they have been infected by the viruses which the vaccine protects against, and if they will therefore have any benefit from it.

The answer is negative because it is considered completely improbable (based on the existing studies) that someone may be infected by all the types of HPV that are covered, especially as regards Gardasil 9. But even if someone has been infected by one type of the vaccine, it has been proven that vaccination reduces the recurrences of infections caused by that specific type.

The only sure way to prevent against infections by specific types of HPV: If a child is vaccinated before starting her/his sexual life, she/he will not be at risk of becoming infected by the HPV types covered by the vaccine.

CHAPTER 3

HPV and the female lower genital tract

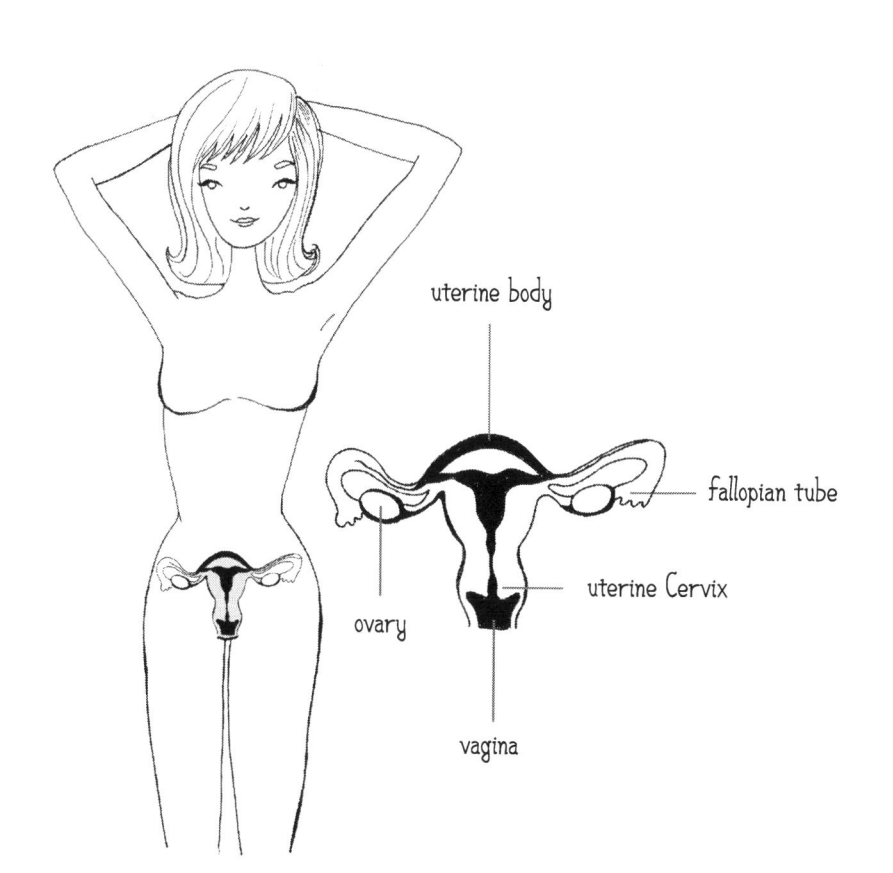

Why are check-ups necessary?

69. In what areas of the female genital organs does HPV cause cancer?

The Figure (p. 97) shows the location of the genital organs in a woman's body.

The female genital organs are: vulva, vagina, uterus (womb), fallopian tubes, and ovaries.

The upper part of the uterus is called the body of the uterus and carries the fetus during pregnancy.

The lower part of the uterus is the cervix. It is a fibromuscular tube that connects the body of the uterus with the vagina.

The uterine cervix dilates during childbirth to allow the fetus to exit.

The female lower genital tract includes the cervix, vagina, and vulva.

The genital types of HPV target the cells of the lower genital tract and the perianal area. The organ in which HPV causes cancer more frequently is the cervix.

70. Why cervical cancer caused by HPV should not worry you if you have regular check-ups

Cancer does not develop overnight and does not appear immediately after the infection.

Ten, twenty or even thirty years may pass between the infection and the appearance of cancer.

Precancerous (premalignant) lesions usually appear before cancer does, and they can be detected and treated.

71. **How long does it take for a precancerous lesion to form?**
    It takes a lot of time, usually years. You therefore have ample time to find them – if there are any – and treat them before it is too late, as long as you get your routine check-ups.

72. **If there are any precancerous lesions, what would be the symptoms?**
    Precancerous lesions caused by HPV have no symptoms and this is why you must have regular check-ups.

73. **Are precancerous lesions visible during a gynecological examination? How are they discovered?**
    Only some precancerous lesions on the vulva are visible. Precancerous lesions on the cervix and the vagina are not visible to the naked eye. They are usually microscopic lesions of the cells and the epithelium. Your physician cannot detect them during a simple gynecological examination.

    This is why your doctor will combine the gynecological examination with a Pap test or an HPV test. If these tests come up with any findings, the next step is usually a colposcopy and a biopsy.

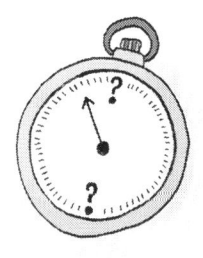

74. **Why should lesions be found while they are still invisible to the naked eye?**

Because cancer can only be prevented during the phase when the cancer cells are contained within the epithelium and have not spread more deeply.

When we talk about precancerous lesions, we mean lesions inside the epithelium (intraepithelial lesions). Under the epithelium there are blood vessels and lymphatic vessels.

If the cancer cells spread under the epithelium, they enter these vessels and travel to other areas of the body, where they 'take residence'. In this case we are talking about metastasis (figures a-h, pp. 160, 161).

WHY YOU SHOULD NOT WORRY ABOUT CERVICAL CANCER, PROVIDED YOU ARE HAVING REGULAR CHECK-UPS:

Before cervical cancer appears, there are usually premalignant lesions which are detected during check-ups.

Don't worry. With the means we have available today (Pap test, HPV test, colposcopy, etc.), you can catch them in time.

Follow your physician's instructions. He knows exactly when and how you must be tested.

HPV hides in the cervix...

Below, I present a short description of the cervical epithelium of the uterine cervix, this being the area that is at a higher risk from HPV. When you read this information, you will get a better understanding of the logic behind check-ups with Pap tests, HPV tests, colposcopies and biopsies.

75. In what type of cervical cells does HPV cause cancer?
It was mentioned previously that your body is covered externally by skin. Your internal organs are covered by mucous membranes. The surface of the skin and the mucosa consists of the epithelium (Figures 2 and 3, p. 50).

On the skin and the mucosa, there are two types of epithelium, the squamous and the glandular epithelium.

The squamous epithelium consists of squamous cells, which form layers (like stones in a stone wall). Their role is mainly protective.

The glandular epithelium is located in the skin's glands (that secrete sweat or smegma) and the mucous glands (responsible for the production of mucus).

As we can see in Figure 8 (p. 102), the uterine cervix is covered in its lower part by two types of epithelium. The part of the cervix that projects into the vagina is covered on its circumference by squamous epithelium, while the endocervical canal and the area around the outer cervical opening are covered by glandular epithelium. The glandular epithelium produces mucus (in larger quantities during ovulation), which the sperm swims in when moving upwards to find the egg.

FIGURE 8: The epithelium infected by HPV on the uterine cervix.
The Figure shows a cross-section of the uterus. We see the cervix in the center. The two different types of epithelium are shown magnified, as we find them on the cervical mucosa: glandular and squamous epithelium.

Transverse section of the uterus (womb)

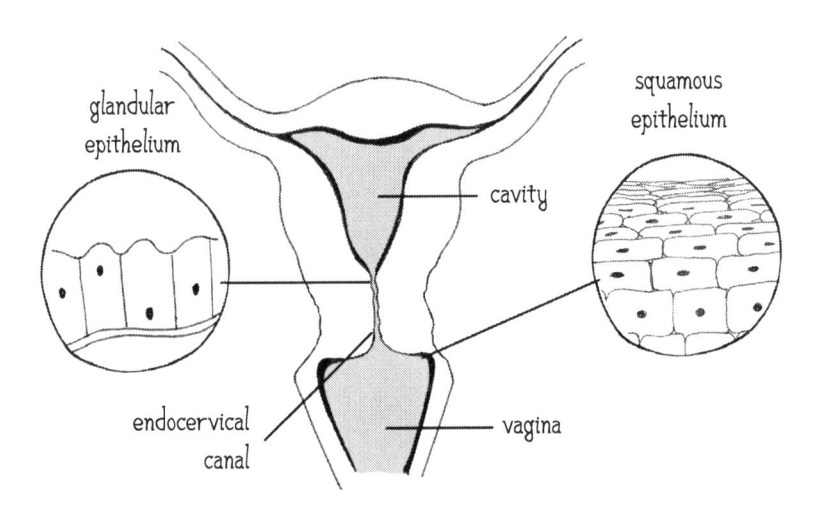

During a woman's reproductive years, a continuous transformation of the glandular epithelium into squamous epithelium is taking place. This process is called metaplasia and the transitional epithelium is called metaplastic epithelium.

The metaplastic epithelium is important because it is the breeding ground for HPV to multiply. The metaplasia process makes it easy for the virus to cause a malignant tumor (this applies only to high-risk HPV). The zone where metaplasia develops is called the transformation zone.

There are two types of cervical cancer, depending on the type of cell they originate from. Squamous cell cancer originates in the squamous epithelium. There is also glandular cell cancer, which originates in the glandular cells of the cervical epithelium. Squamous cell cancer is the most common one, and usually starts inside the metaplastic epithelium of the transformation zone.

76. How do we find precancerous lesions in the cervix?

As mentioned before, precancerous lesions are not visible to the naked eye during a gynecological examination. They are detected during an examination with magnifying instruments, like the colposcope and microscope. This is why you must have regular Pap tests and/or HPV tests.

The doctor collects cells from the surface of the cervix, which are then examined under the microscope (Pap test). Approximately 2-5% of women have a Pap test with cell changes due to HPV at any one screening.

If abnormal cells are discovered, you must then have a colposcopy.

During a colposcopy, the surface of the uterine cervix is examined in detail with the help of a colposcope (an instrument with magnifying lens, like the microscope), suspicious areas are identified, and biopsies are taken (small tissue samples).

These biopsies are then examined under a microscope (histological examination). During histological examination, both the morphology of the cells and the structure of the epithelium of the excised tissue are examined.

The HPV test (carried out like the Pap-test) seeks to identify any oncogenic types of HPV. If the result is positive, the same process that was described above (after an abnormal Pap test) is followed in most cases (colposcopy, biopsies).

The final diagnosis is made after studying the results of all these tests (gynecological examination, Pap test, HPV test, colposcopy, and biopsy).

There are cases where, in order to exclude invasive cancer, further testing is required by curettage of the endocervical canal, or by removal of part of the cervix (cone biopsy). The procedure will be decided by your doctor based on the particularity of your case.

You will find more details in the following pages of the book.

CHAPTER 4

Pap test

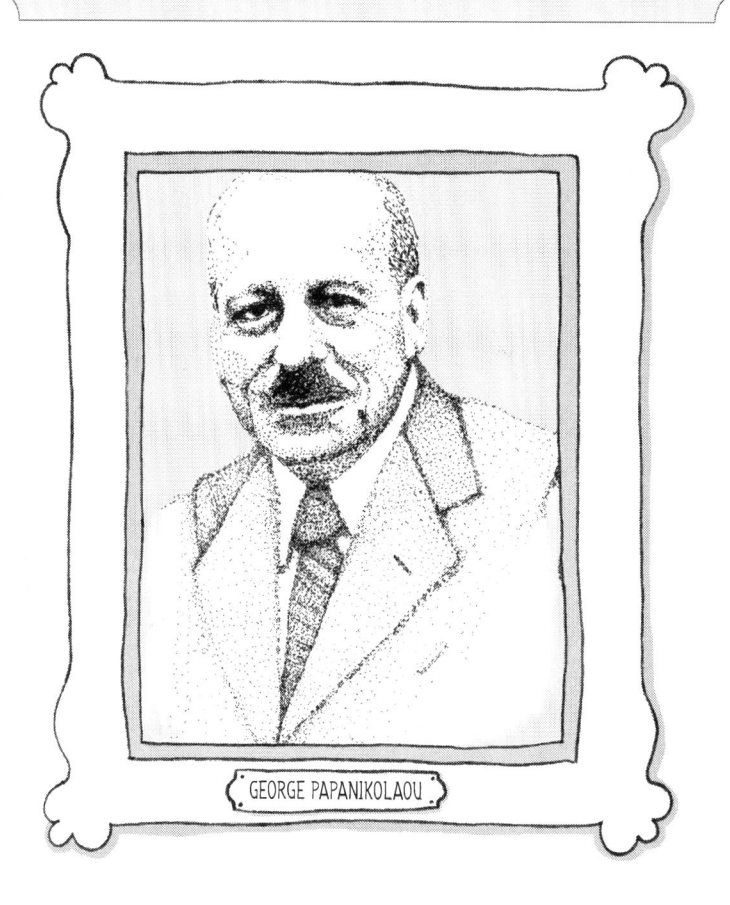

GEORGE PAPANIKOLAOU

Georgios Papanikolaou

Born in 1883 in Greece, he graduated from the Medical School of the University of Athens, Greece. He continued with post-graduate studies and a PhD in Germany. He returned to Greece and fought in the Balkan Wars in 1912-13. He then immigrated with his wife to the USA and was hired by Cornell University in 1914. In 1928 he published his first paper on the early diagnosis of cancer. In 1941 he published his findings on the value of studying cells from vaginal and cervical smears and in 1943 he published, together with Trauth, his classic and famous study that established the preventive examination of cervical and vaginal smears for the early diagnosis of cervical cancer.

Population screening was immediately implemented in the USA, also spreading to Europe after 1960.

In 1954 he published the Atlas of Exfoliative Cytology, which is considered a monumental opus, where techniques for studying cells from various body organs are described. He visited Greece in 1957 and received many honors.

Papanikolaou had the satisfaction of seeing his work recognized on a global scale during his lifetime. He had received countless expressions of gratitude and had been honored internationally with many awards and distinctions. In 1961, he was appointed Director of the Anticancer Research Institute that was founded in Miami, Florida, which was given his name. He worked until the last days of his life. He died of a heart attack in 1962.

PAP TEST

77. What is the Pap test?
In the mid-20th century, George Papanikolaou invented the Pap smear. He discovered that, by collecting cells from the surface of the mucosa and studying them under the microscope, you can identify lesions that are hiding inside the epithelium.

The method became internationally known as the «Pap test» and has saved millions of lives from cervical cancer.

78. How is the Pap test performed?
The woman sits in the gynecological chair, like she does during a gynecological examination. The doctor inserts the speculum inside the vagina and opens the vaginal canal to reveal the uterine cervix. A soft brush that looks like a tiny broom is brushed around the surface of the cervix and the endocervical canal, collecting cells. The test doesn't hurt. It may cause mild crampy discomfort for the patient. These cells are later stained and evaluated through a microscope (Figure 9, p. 108).

79. What do we mean by a negative Pap test?
A negative Pap test means that no abnormal cells were found.

80. Can a Pap test come out negative and miss a lesion?
Yes, that's possible, because the cells are collected from the surface of the mucous membranes, and these are not always representative of the lesions inside the epithelium layers.

81. **Is it possible to have more serious lesions than what the Pap test showed?**
    Yes, it is possible, for the reason mentioned in the previous question, but also because perhaps no cells were collected from the worse-off area.

82. **What is the reliability of the Pap test?**
    It ranges between 50-75%, in regards to detecting precancerous lesions.

FIGURE 9: Pap test
Cervical cells are collected with a brush. They are then stored in a special vial and are later examined under a microscope.

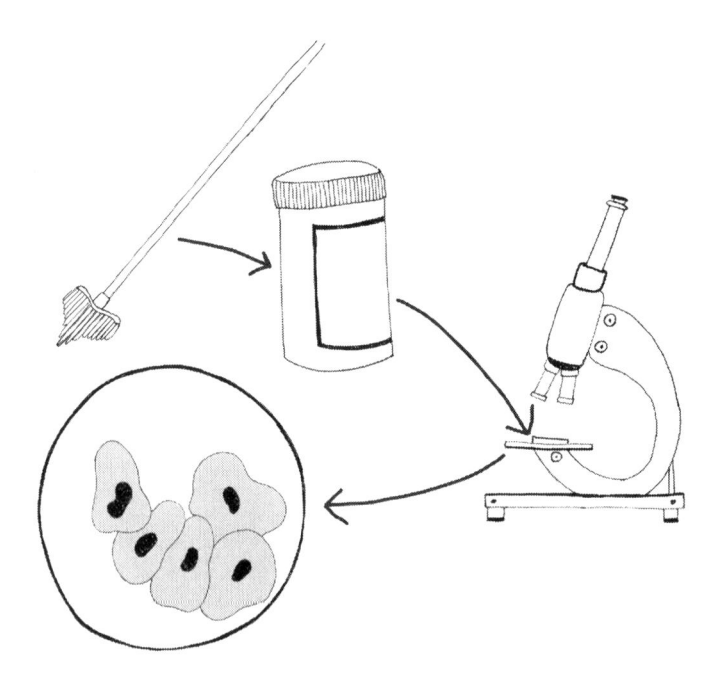

83. How can the reliability of the Pap test be improved?

If we want to reduce the risk of missing a precancerous lesion:

- The Pap test must be repeated at regular intervals. This significantly reduces the probability of missing cancer, because carcinogenesis in the cervix is usually a drawn out process (carcinogenesis is the process by which normal cells are transformed into cancer cells). Even if a lesion is missed in one Pap test, it is considered improbable that it will be missed in three successive tests.
- A second way is to combine the Pap test with an HPV test. The HPV test, which is described in the next chapter, detects the viral load from oncogenic types of HPV. This method is more costly than the Pap test alone but offers a higher than 90% reliability in detecting precancerous lesions.

84. What can the examination of the cervical cells under the microscope show?

After you get the results of your Pap test, you may see the following results:

- Normal cells
- Inflammatory lesions from causes other than HPV (chlamydia, etc.) or atrophic lesions
- Cells with infection from HPV (LSIL category)
- Cells with precancerous lesions (HSIL category) or cells suspect for cancer of the squamous or glandular epithelium
- Cells with lesions that cannot be assessed with precision (ASCUS category)

85. **If the Pap test shows inflammation or atrophy, what happens next?**

The main purpose of the Pap test is to prevent cervical cancer. We are, therefore, primarily interested in detecting any atypical cells.

Often, an examination under the microscope may diagnose inflammations from several microorganisms (bacteria, fungi, trichomoniasis, etc). These findings simply help your doctor to prescribe a treatment if they find it necessary.

Also, in menopausal women, test results frequently show atrophic lesions of the epithelium. This is due to the drop in estrogen levels during menopause.

Sometimes, due to severe inflammation or atrophy of the epithelium, the results from the cytological lab mention that it is not possible to correctly evaluate the test, and that it needs to be repeated. In such a case, treatment is prescribed, and after a certain period the Pap test is repeated, or an HPV test is also done.

86. **If the Pap test shows abnormal cells, what is their significance and what are the next steps to be taken?**

If a Pap test discovers cells suspect for precancerous lesions or cancer (Figure 10, p. 111), the next step is a colposcopy and biopsies. When LSIL or HSIL lesions are found by a Pap test, or there is suspicion for cancer, the next step is a colposcopy.

With regard to the ASCUS category, your doctor may recommend an HPV test. If it is positive for oncogenic types of HPV, you must then undergo a colposcopy.

FIGURE 10: Pap smear with cervical cells
1. Normal cells
2. Cells with an HPV infection
3. Precancerous cells

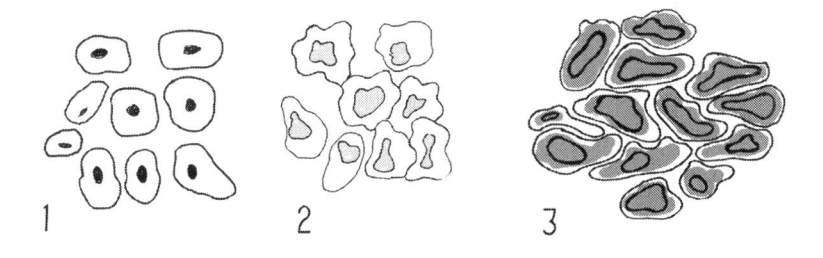

In any case, you must consult your doctor. They will offer appropriate guidance. Each woman's needs must be addressed on an individual basis.

Below, we list some general rules based on the general recommendations by the American Society for Colposcopy and Cervical Pathology about the importance of each Pap test diagnosis and how the result should be managed.

ASC: This group includes ASCUS and ASC-H. ASCUS means Atypical Squamous Cells of Undetermined Significance. Between 2-10% of cases will have this Pap interpretation. Some atypical squamous epithelial cells are found, without, however, being able to accurately determine the severity. There are two subcategories of ASC: ASCUS and ASC-H (Atypical Squamous Cells – cannot rule out High-grade).

If there is an ASCUS result, milder lesions are usually presumed, without excluding more serious ones. Approximately 50-60% of women having this Pap reading are entirely normal (HPV negative and no cervical disease), and 40-50% are High-Risk HPV positive, with half of those having detectable cervical changes due to HPV (mostly LSIL). Approximately 6-9% will have high-grade changes (HSIL, CIN2 or 3) and, rarely, cervical cancer (approximately 1/1000 ASC-US).

Classifying the test as ASC-H means that the existence of a more serious lesion is possible. Some cells are abnormal enough to be suggestive, but not definitive, of a high-grade lesion. Between 60-80% of women with ASC-H test positive for high-risk HPV, and the risk of CIN2,3+ is much higher than that of ASC-US.

AGUS: This means that atypical glandular cells were found, but there cannot be a precise diagnosis. This diagnosis is found in 0.2-0.8% of the general population. In 50-70% of these cases, further testing will show that there is no problem, and that it was a simple overestimation. However, in the greatest part of the rest of the women, further testing will show, in order of frequency: HSIL, adenocarcinoma in situ (non-metastatic) and, in a few cases, invasive cancer. The more advanced the age, the greater the risk for finding more severe lesions. There are cases (usually in women older than 35), where the doctor will ask to check the endometrium, apart from the cervix, fearing adenocarcinoma of the endometrium.

LSIL: This means cells with low-grade lesions. They are found in over 3% of the Pap tests in ages above 30, but in much higher percentages if we focus on younger ages. If all the women whose Pap tests showed LSIL are checked with a colposcopy and biopsy, we will find that the final diagnosis is HSIL in around 10% of these women.

HSIL: This means cells with high-grade lesions. In the general population we see this result in only 0.3-0.8% of the tests. With further examination (colposcopy), which is imperative in this case, high-grade lesions are usually found. In a few cases the final diagnosis is LSIL (usually cases that were overestimated during the cytological evaluation). There are, however, a few cases where the test shows HSIL and, after the examination, the final diagnosis is invasive cancer (1-4%). Special attention must be given to women above 30 years of age when the Pap test shows HSIL.

87. Is any preparation necessary before a Pap test?

As we described above, during a Pap test cells are collected from the surface of the cervix. For this reason, it is better not to get the test during menstruation, because the menstruation blood will have washed away cells from the cervical surface.

Two days before the test the woman must not have any vaginal douches or use intravaginal creams.

It is also recommended not to have sex 24 hours prior to the test.

88. At what age should women start getting Pap tests?

From the age of 21 (recommendation of the American College of Obstetricians and Gynecologists - 2013).

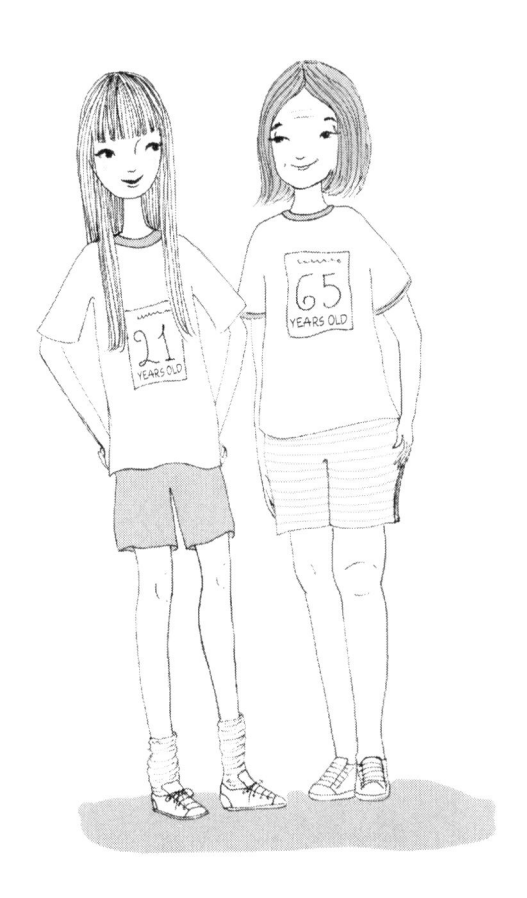

89. **Up to what age should women keep getting Pap tests?**
    Up to the age of 65. Women with a history of precancerous lesions or cancer of the lower genital tract must continue to be tested after the age of 65.

90. **Should women get Pap tests during pregnancy?**
    If it has been a long time since they last had a Pap test, it would be better to get one. Usually, the first set of tests

during a pregnancy is a good opportunity for a Pap test, especially for women who had not had regular check-ups in the past.

A Pap test is not dangerous to pregnancy.

91. Should women who are not sexually active at present have a Pap test?

They may have contracted one or more oncogenic types of HPV in the past and not be aware of it. Therefore, it is recommended that they are tested.

92. Should women who have had a hysterectomy get Pap tests?

If the hysterectomy was done because of malignancy, follow-ups with Pap tests are necessary, should any lesions appear in the vagina. The same applies to cases with a history of premalignant (precancerous) lesions on the cervix in the past or in any case where the hysterectomy was performed for another reason (e.g. fibromyomas, hemorrhage, endometriosis), but premalignant lesions were found on the cervix during the histological examination.

If there was a subtotal hysterectomy for benign diseases (only the body of the uterus was removed and the cervix remains), they must certainly continue to have Pap tests like the rest of the population.

Only in those cases where there was a total hysterectomy (the cervix was also removed) for a benign disease and there is no history of HPV infection, is it recommended to discontinue the cytological tests of the vagina.

CHAPTER 5

HPV test

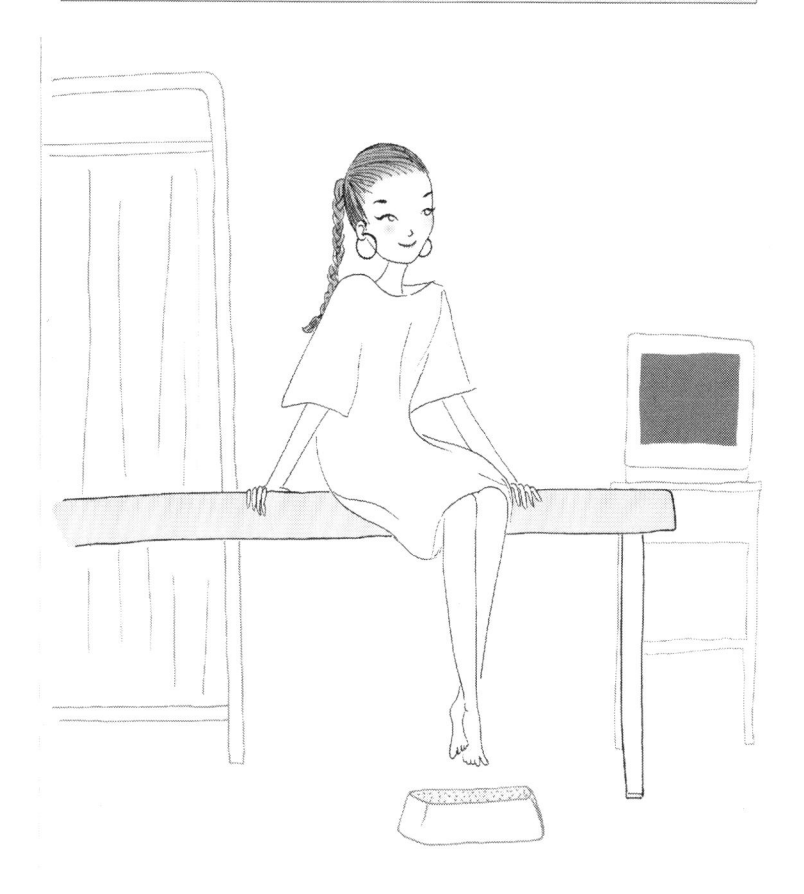

93. What is the HPV test?

This is a test that informs us whether there are oncogenic types of HPV in the cells of your cervix, at a quantity (virus load) that signifies the existence of HPV infection.

The HPV test is used in the prevention of cervical cancer.

94. What is the logic behind the HPV test?

It has been proven that carcinogenesis in the cervix usually starts after a persistent or recurring infection by oncogenic types of HPV. The HPV test detects this infection.

95. How is the HPV test performed?

Material is collected from the cervix in the same manner as in the Pap test (by preserving the material in a special liquid) as seen in Figure 9, p. 108.

Pap test	HPV TEST
Detects atypical cells on the uterine cervix	Detects infection from oncogenic types of HPV on the uterine cervix

96. Can an HPV test be performed together with the Pap test?

It can be performed together with the Pap test, in which case the check-up is considered even more reliable (the combination of the two tests is called a "double test or co-testing") (Figure 11, p. 119).

If either of these two tests comes up with suspect results, a colposcopy is recommended. The colposcopy identifies suspect areas and biopsies are taken.

FIGURE 11: What do the Pap test and HPV test detect?
The Pap test detects atypical cells, and the HPV test detects DNA of oncogenic types of HPV.

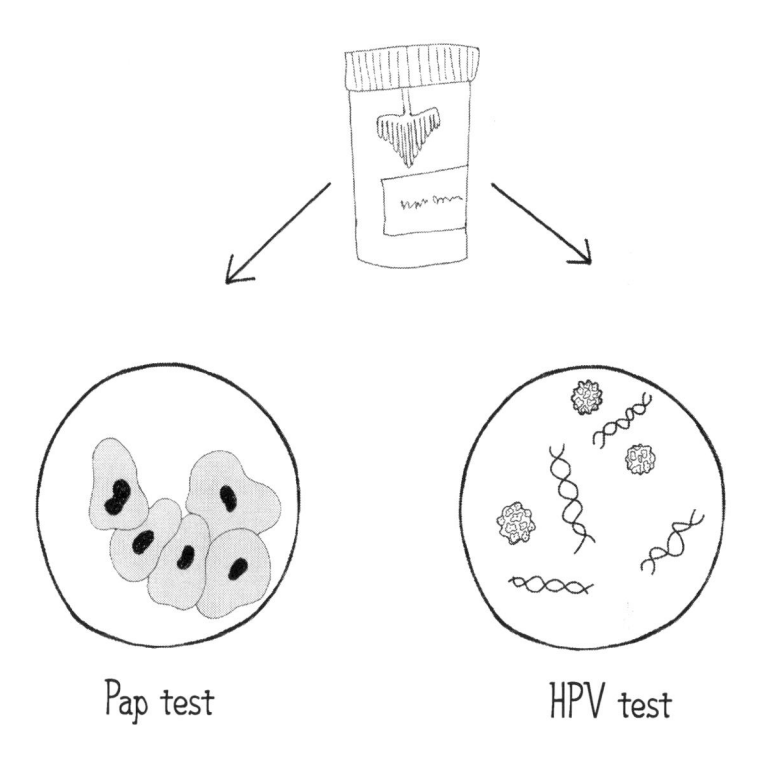

Pap test   HPV test

97. At what age is it recommended that women get an HPV test and why?

Infection with HPV is common in younger women, due to the frequent change of sexual partners. Cancer is rare in this age group. For this reason, when it comes to population screening, scientific societies across the world recommend that all women 30 years of age and older get HPV tests. Younger women are screened by Pap tests.

98. **If the HPV test comes out positive, does this mean that you have something serious?**
Not always. Most times, especially in young ages, it is a simple infection. But there are some cases where precancerous lesions might be present.

99. **What is the reliability of the HPV test and the double test?**
The reliability of the HPV test in detecting precancerous lesions is 92%. The reliability increases even more if combined with a Pap test (the combination of the two is called a double test).

Your doctor will choose, depending on your age and history, which test you must have (Pap or HPV) or if you need to have both tests together. Also, they will decide if you need a colposcopy or biopsy or something else.

100. **How should a woman prepare before an HPV test?**
Preparation is the same as that described for the Pap test, in question 87, p. 113.

101. **Are there HPV tests that show the type of the virus?**
Yes, there are HPV tests which inform us whether there is an infection, especially by HPV 16, HPV 18 or another oncogenic type of HPV.

102. **Are there different types of HPV tests?**
Yes, there are. They are produced by different companies, but are based on the same philosophy. It is, of course, recommended that only tests that have been thoroughly tested and with a proven reliability are used. Both Eu-

ropean and American scientific societies and organizations (such as the FDA) issue related announcements regarding the tests that are approved for use.

103. What are the possible results of the HPV test and what do they mean?
- Negative: It means that no oncogenic types of HPV were found.
- Positive: Oncogenic types of HPV were detected.
- Positive for a specific type (HPV 16 or HPV 18).

104. In what cases in general are HPV tests recommended?
The HPV test is recommended for the screening of asymptomatic women (aged >30 years) in combination with a Pap test or on its own. The HPV test is used in other cases as well, such as:
- For the follow-up of patients after the surgical removal of precancerous lesions and
- To further check ambiguous cytological findings of the Pap test (e.g. ASCUS category).

DON'T FORGET

The role of the HPV test is to detect an infection by oncogenic types of HPV.

CHAPTER 6

Colposcopy – Biopsy

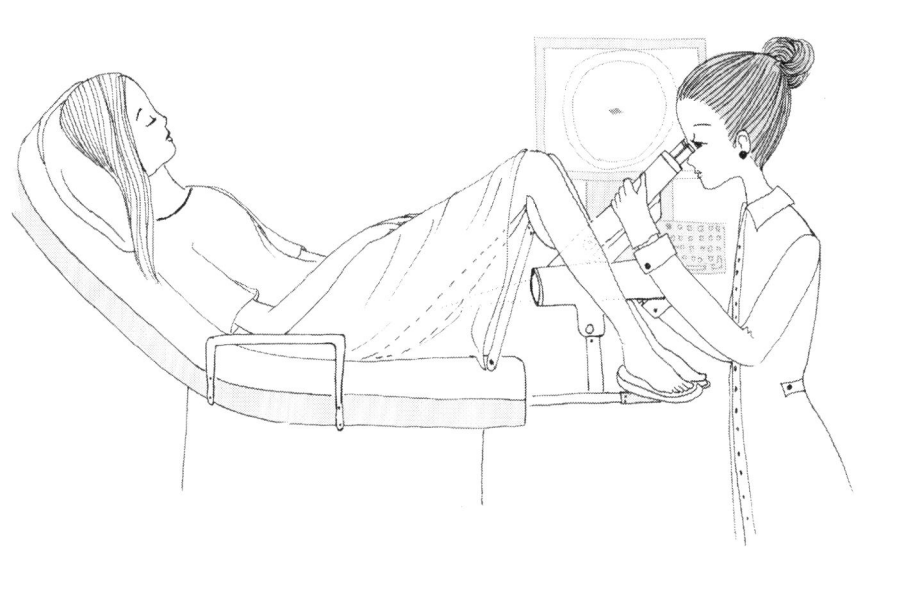

Colposcopy

105. What is a colposcope?

The colposcope looks like a microscope. Its lenses magnify the image multiple times. The person looking through the colposcope can magnify the area that interests him multiple times (8, 12, 20, or even 30 times). The colposcope also has a strong light fitted onto it, which is adjusted by the user, as well as special green and blue filters that help its user identify details.

The colposcope was invented by Hans Hinselmann, from Germany, who started using it in 1924 to detect cancerous lesions on the cervix.

Today, the colposcope is used to locate precancerous lesions and cancer in the lower genital tract and the perianal area.

106. What is a colposcopy?

A colposcopy is an examination of the skin and mucous membranes of the lower genital tract (cervix, vagina and vulva) through a colposcope. As seen on the image of the previous page, the woman lies on the examination chair, exactly like she does during a pelvic examination. Through a colposcope, your doctor directly examines your cervix, vagina, and vulva under magnification.

The perianal area and the anal canal are also examined with the help of a colposcope. This examination is called a high-resolution anoscopy, which is different than a simple anoscopy.

107. What is the colposcopy used for?

Colposcopes are very useful in identifying precancerous lesions and cancer.

A colposcopy helps us locate suspect areas – which are not visible to a naked eye examination – and if deemed necessary, take biopsies (small tissue samples).

It is also useful for defining transformation zones, which are the most frequent areas where normal cells are transformed into cancer cells in the cervix, and to determine our next steps (diagnostic or surgical).

The role of a colposcopy is to correctly guide the doctor in deciding which area to take the biopsies from or how to plan the removal of a wider area, with the main aim of not missing invasive cancer.

108. Is a colposcope used during surgery?

A colposcope is also used in surgery during special procedures. For example, in the LEEP procedure (see question 195, p. 172) the surgeon overviews the operating field through a colposcope. This allows him to magnify the field in which he is operating and also provides better lighting, in order to remove the area with the lesions with the greatest precision possible.

There is also the option of connecting a colposcope to a carbon dioxide laser device. With the help of a special control pad, the doctor directs the laser on the lesion with millimeter accuracy.

109. When is a colposcopy recommended?
A colposcopy is recommended in the following cases:
- If suspect cells are found by a Pap test.
- If the HPV test is positive (this means that there is an infection from oncogenic types of HPV).
- When the doctor sees something suspicious during a simple examination.
- Before several procedures in the lower genital tract to assess the extent of the lesions.

110. How is a colposcopy performed?
The woman lies in the gynecological examination position. A colposcope is placed at a small distance (10-15 cm) from her body. The doctor, using the strong light and magnification provided by the colposcope, examines in detail the skin and mucous membranes.

A solution of diluted acetic acid (similar to white vinegar) is used for the colposcopy. By applying this solution on the skin and mucous membranes, lesions that were not visible up to then are revealed.

It is possible, if the doctor finds it necessary, to use an iodine solution (called lugol).

111. Are biopsies always performed during a colposcopy?
No, they are not. In some cases the doctor will decide that they are not necessary.

In other cases, when the lesions found are very serious and cover a large area, the doctor knows that they cannot count on isolated biopsies and that they must surgically remove a larger area in order to exclude invasive cancer (which may not be visible during the colposcopy).

112. Are the colposcopy and biopsies painful?

The acetic acid solution used during the colposcopy causes a mild burning sensation, which quickly subsides.

Special instruments (biopsy forceps) are used for taking biopsies from the cervix, which are not painful. Patients feel only a slight discomfort, and no painkillers are necessary.

113. Does the colposcopy have any risk?

No. If you are allergic to iodine you must tell your doctor not to use any iodine solution.

If you also get a biopsy, it is recommended that you abstain from any sexual activity for 3-4 days. If after the biopsy you have any vaginal discharge with blood, it is recommended that you abstain from sex for a week.

114. Can you get a colposcopy during pregnancy?

Yes, you can, if there is a relevant indication, e.g. an abnormal Pap test. Biopsies may also be performed if deemed necessary.

115. Is any preparation necessary before a colposcopy?

- You must make your appointment on a day when you do not have your period.
- If there is any inflammation in the lower genital tract (cervix, vagina, vulva), it would be best to get treatment before the colposcopy. Therefore, if you have symptoms and suspect anything like that, consult your doctor.
- Remember to have with you the results of any previous tests (Pap test, HPV test, etc.).

116. How reliable is a colposcopy?

A colposcopy is a subjective examination. It goes without saying that it must be performed by a well-trained doctor. The accuracy of the diagnosis depends on many parameters. The doctor takes into consideration the findings of the other tests, as well as the patient's history. In cases where there is a risk of missing cancer (for example when the Pap test shows precancerous lesions – HSIL and extensive lesions are visible during the colposcopy), it is necessary not to rely only on what one sees in the colposcopy and isolated biopsies, but also to remove part of the cervix.

Colposcopic biopsy

117. What exactly is a colposcopic biopsy and how is it performed?

We described before how we collect cells only from the surface of the epithelium when taking a Pap test.

During a biopsy, we remove a small piece of tissue with special forceps (Figure 12, p. 129). We can thus study under the microscope the entire thickness of the epithelium as well as the area under the epithelium, to diagnose with precision whether it is a precancerous lesion or cancer.

118. Why do we perform biopsies?

A biopsy is performed to exclude precancerous lesions or cancer. Only a biopsy can provide an accurate diagnosis of the excised tissue pathology.

FIGURE 12: Biopsy

We see the part of the removed tissue (epithelium and the underlying stroma) that is later examined under the microscope.

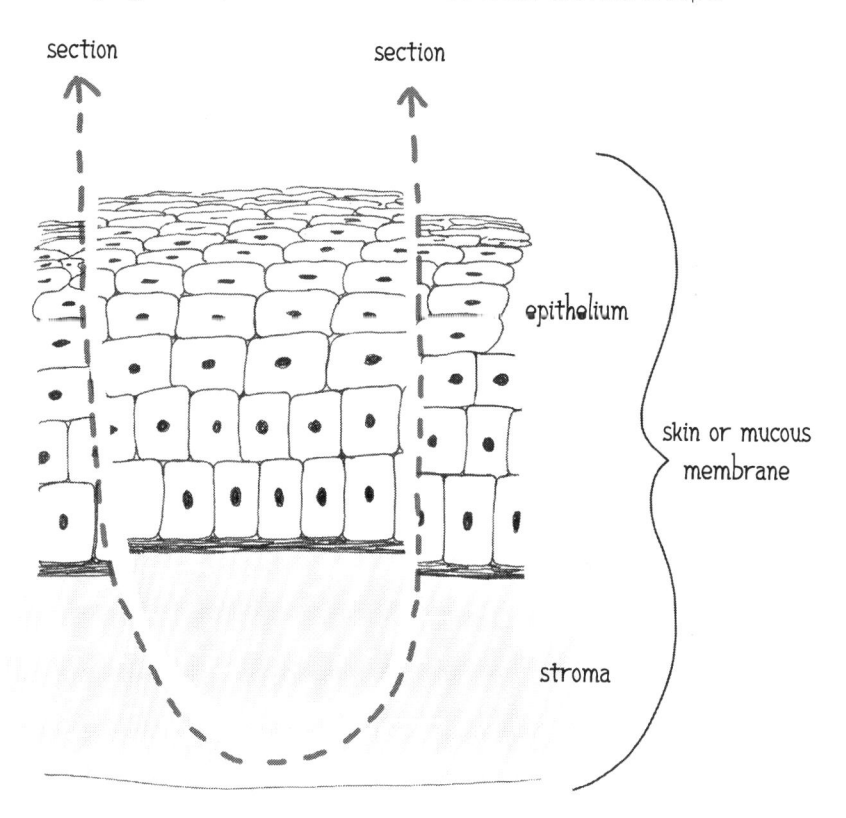

119. What is the reliability of a biopsy taken during a colposcopy?

This question can be rephrased. Can a biopsy not show the problem?

A colposcopic biopsy is reliable, on condition that it is taken from the right location.

There is the human subjective factor, which has partly to do with the doctor's experience. There are, however, limits, because only the surface of the epithelium is examined during a colposcopy.

The doctor knows their limits and the limits of the examination, and will give you the right advice.

120. What does the doctor see under the microscope when examining a biopsy?

They see the epithelium and the area under the epithelium, called stroma (Figure 12, p. 129).

They examine the morphology of the cells and the structure of the epithelium.

121. What is the difference between a biopsy and a Pap test?

The histological examination of a biopsy will show the entire pathology of the tissue removed (all layers of the epithelium are examined, as well as the tissue under the basal membrane, called stroma).

During a Pap test we only collect cells from the surface of the epithelium. The cells that are examined are not always representative of the severity of the lesions inside the tissue.

122. What are the possible diagnoses after a cervical biopsy?

The possible diagnoses are:
- Normal epithelium
- Infection of the epithelium by HPV
- Precancerous lesion
- Invasive cancer

123. How do we get from a check-up to a biopsy?

A check-up usually includes a pelvic examination, a Pap test or HPV test, or both. The significance of the results of the check-up is shown in Table 4.

The doctor takes into consideration your history, age, and the results of the Pap test or HPV test.

As mentioned above, in most cases with abnormal findings, the next step is a colposcopy.

Whether biopsies will be taken or not will be assessed during the colposcopy.

If there are any serious lesions, your doctor may not rely only on isolated biopsies, but tell you that they must remove part of the cervix (usually if there is fear that there is an underlying cancer starting).

You must consult a doctor experienced on this subject (colposcopy specialist).

TABLE 4

What the results of your routine check-up may show

Test	HPV/DNA Test	Pap test	
Result	Positive	Cell infection from HPV	Abnormal (atypical) cells
Significance	There is infection from high-risk types of HPV or precancerous lesion.	Usually simple infection. Small possibility of precancerous lesion.	Suspicion of possible precancerous lesion or cancer

CHAPTER 7
Benign diseases caused by genital types of HPV

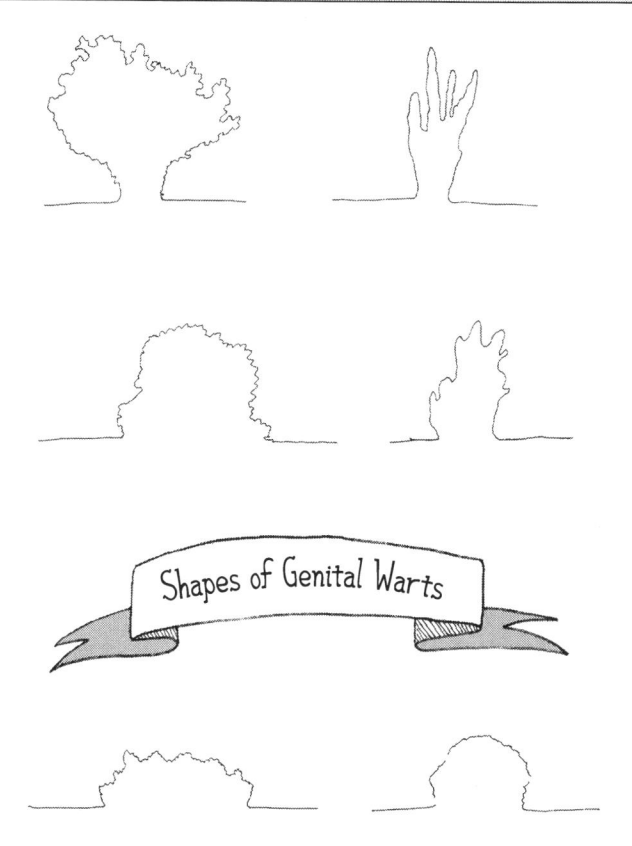

Shapes of Genital Warts

Subclinical lesions on the skin and mucous membranes

124. What are subclinical lesions caused by HPV?
As we described in chapter one (questions 11-13, pp. 57-61, Figure 7, p. 62), HPV causes infections of the skin and mucous membranes. Most of them cause no symptoms and are not visible to the naked eye. Not even your doctor can see them while examining you without any magnifying devices. This is where the name «subclinical lesions» came from, meaning invisible during a clinical examination.

125. How frequent are subclinical lesions caused by HPV?
Most people are infected with certain genital types of HPV during sexual intercourse and get subclinical infections caused by HPV on the skin and mucous membranes of the genital organs, during certain phases of their life.

The chances of becoming infected with HPV and developing subclinical lesions are proportional to the number of sexual partners. The sexual history of each partner and the use of a condom also play an important role.

126. What is the incidence of subclinical lesions caused by HPV in the general population compared to the incidence of genital warts?
The incidence of subclinical lesions is many times higher than the incidence of genital warts. The latter is calculated at 1-3% of individuals who have not been vaccinated.

127. Do subclinical lesions cause symptoms? How are they discovered?

No, they cause no symptoms and can only be found with magnifying instruments, like the colposcope or microscope (with a Pap-test and biopsies). Another way to identify a subclinical infection is to test directly for the virus DNA (e.g. taking an HPV test from the cervix).

128. What types of HPV cause subclinical lesions?

All genital types of HPV (low and high-risk) cause subclinical lesions.

129. What is the prognosis for subclinical lesions caused by HPV?

Those subclinical lesions that are caused by low-risk types of HPV usually clear spontaneously within one year.
- As for subclinical lesions caused by high-risk types of HPV:
- 70% are suppressed within one year by the immune system
- 90% are suppressed within 3 years by the immune system

In 10% of the cases, the immune system cannot suppress the infection caused by an oncogenic type of HPV. The infection persists or is temporarily suppressed and recurs later. In these cases there is an increased risk for mutations and appearance of premalignant (precancerous) lesions initially and then cancer.

130. If an infection by a cancer-causing type of HPV is discovered what is the next step?
The next step is usually a colposcopy, to look for premalignant lesions, if there are any.

131. What is the treatment for subclinical lesions?
No treatment is recommended, since, as mentioned above, most of these infections clear spontaneously.

132. Which subclinical lesions do we follow up and why?
Infections caused by oncogenic types of HPV require closer follow-up due to the risk for precancerous lesions and cancer. There is a higher risk when HPVs 16 and 18 are found.

Genital warts

A) What are genital warts, what causes them and how will you recognize them?

133. What are genital warts?
Genital warts are benign tumors that protrude from the skin and the mucous membranes of the lower genital tract and the anal area. This is a sexually transmitted viral disease.

134. What causes genital warts?
Genital warts are caused by specific types of HPV. The infection of the skin and mucous membranes results in hy-

perplasia (thickening) of the epithelium and the formation of the characteristic warty (condylomatous) lesions.

135. What do genital warts look like?

Warts are usually visible to a naked eye examination. They protrude from the skin and are palpable. They are most commonly felt as raised bumps, but they may be so small that they often go unnoticed. Most of them are small in size (less than one centimeter). In some cases, however, they are larger than one centimeter.

Warts have many different shapes. (see shapes of warts, p. 133)

Their color varies. They may be skin-colored or lighter (nearly white). Some warts are darker than the skin (more brown or gray). Genital warts on the mucosa (inside the labia, the vagina, cervix, and inside the anal canal) are pink or whitish.

136. Is it a common disease?

It is estimated that the probability of a woman getting genital warts during her lifetime is around 1-3%. The possibility of genital warts is related to the number of sexual partners. Warts are more common in individuals with multiple sexual partners or high-risk sexual partners (who have a history of many sexual partners). This, of course, does not mean that there aren't people with genital warts who report a single sexual partner.

137. Where do warts appear in women?

In women, warts appear in the vulva, perineum, pubic area, vagina, cervix, urethra, the perianal area and the anal canal (Figure 13, p. 138).

FIGURE 13: The external genital organs of a woman

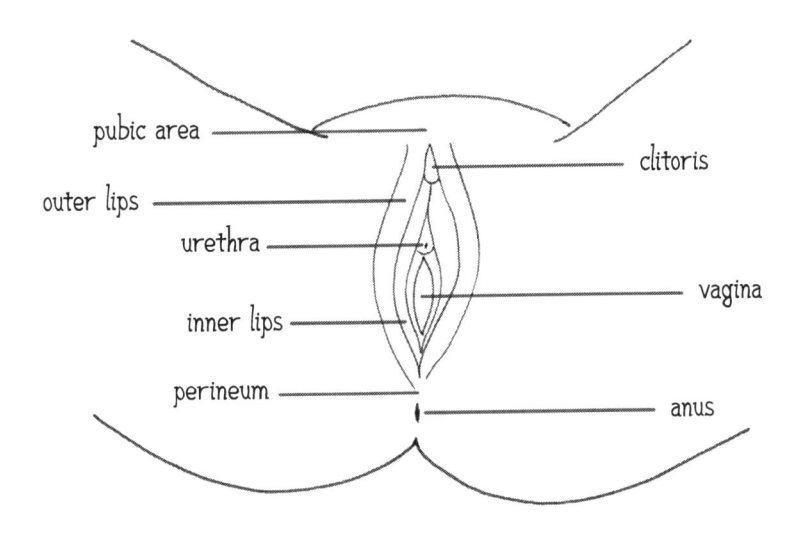

- pubic area
- outer lips
- urethra
- inner lips
- perineum
- clitoris
- vagina
- anus

138. Where do warts appear in men?

Usually on the penis. In uncircumcised men, they are more frequent on the glans (head) of the penis. Less frequently, they are found on the pubis, scrotum, groin and the perianal area. Anal warts are more frequent in receptive homosexuals, and the anal canal must be checked. A few cases of perianal warts have also been found in men and women who did not report any anal intercourse.

139. Is the appearance of warts in the mouth frequent?

No, it is not. Warts in the genital area and the anus are more common, because vaginal and anal intercourse entail more intense friction (rubbing).

140. What types of HPV cause genital warts?

Around 90% of genital warts are caused by HPV 6 and 11. In the rest of the cases other types are also detected (also high-risk, such as HPV 16).

More specifically, in patients with warts we also occasionally detect HPV 16, 18, 31, 33 and 35. There is usually a parallel infection with high-risk types of HPV, which means a future risk for precancerous lesions.

B) Transmission of genital warts

141. How are genital warts transmitted?

Genital warts are mainly transmitted through sexual contact and are classified as sexually transmitted diseases.

If the skin and mucous membranes of your genital organs are rubbed with the skin or mucous membranes of an infected individual, the virus enters your epithelium and may start causing infection.

The most common ways of transmission are vaginal and anal intercourse. Transmission through oral sex and rubbing of the genital area with infected fingers or sex toys is also possible.

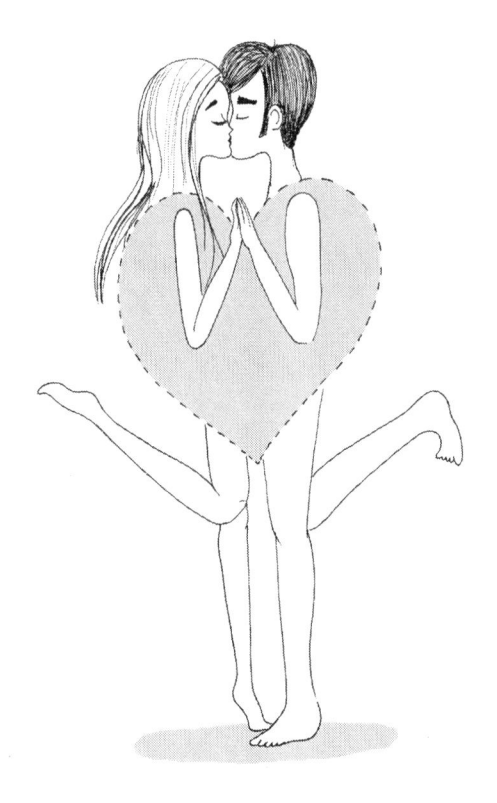

142. If you have intercourse with an infected individual is infection inevitable?

Your immune system may not allow the virus to cause extensive infection. In many people, the initial infection caused by HPV is spontaneously suppressed by their defense system and they are not even aware that they were infected, because they never had any visible lesions or symptoms.

If you have intercourse with an individual with visible genital warts, the possibility that you will get warts within the next six months is 60-70%.

143. How long after the infection do genital warts appear?

Usually it takes a few weeks or up to several months from the day of the infection until visible lesions appear (4 weeks to 8 months).

You may, however, be infected and never get visible warts. In rare cases, warts may appear years after the infection. HPV can remain latent in some people for years or decades before developing warts or cervical disease.

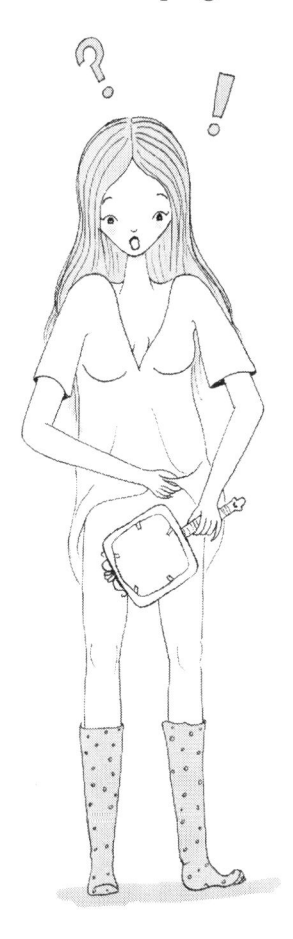

In these cases we presume that something went wrong with the immune system and the virus was re-activated.

It is not possible to determine exactly when, or from whom, an individual contracted the virus.

144. How can you know if the individual you will have intercourse with has the infection and that you may become infected?

You cannot always know. There is certainty only if this person has genital warts at the moment.

They may also have been infected in the past and carry HPV in their cells.

145. What are your chances of contracting genital warts from a partner?

- If your partner has visible warts at the present time, it is highly possible that you will become infected (60-70%) because a large viral load is transmitted during each sexual contact.
- If your partner has had genital warts recently, and it is less than 6 months since they were treated, it is possible that you will become infected, because there are still lesions that are not visible to the naked eye. These lesions slowly subside on their own, usually within the next 6-12 months, but in some cases remain for 2-3 years.
- There is always a chance of becoming infectious again because of a recurrence of an old infection from HPV. No one can know exactly when this might happen. However, the more time passes since treatment of the last wart, the less infectious one is considered.

- If at this time an old infection of your partner has recurred and their lesions are not visible, they may be transmitting their infection to you without either of you being aware of it.

146. How can you find out when and who infected you?

From the above (question 145) it is clear that you cannot accurately know when and who infected you.

147. If someone has common warts, can they infect you with genital warts?

No. The HPV types that cause common warts are different from those that cause genital warts (they don't belong to the genital types of HPV).

148. How can we explain genital warts in areas where there is no friction during sexual intercourse?

People with genital warts frequently get them in other areas, such as the pubis, groin, and elsewhere. The shaving or hair removal of these areas sometimes causes small abrasions, which offer HPV the opportunity to enter and infect the basal layer of the epithelium. Also, rubbing or scratching an area (such as e.g. the anus), with infected fingers-fingernails can cause new lesions to appear.

149. If a woman gets genital warts, must her partner be examined?

If a woman gets genital warts, we recommend that her partner is also examined as a precaution. Men who observe any changes on their penis are also advised to get checked. We don't recommend a routine check-up for all men simply because their partner was found with an HPV infection in her Pap test.

C) Diagnosis of genital warts

150. What are the symptoms of genital warts?
Genital warts don't hurt and usually cause no symptoms. There are people who discover them by chance. Sometimes, they cause itching.

151. How does a woman discover genital warts?
Genital warts protrude from the skin, are visible, and are usually palpable. Women may discover genital warts on their pubis, vulva, perineum, and perianal area.

152. How can you know if you have genital warts elsewhere?
After your doctor examines you, they can tell you if you have genital warts in the vagina, cervix or inside the anal canal.

153. What is the association between genital warts and cancers caused by HPV?
Precancerous lesions in the anal canal and genital area are more frequent in women with genital warts or a history of genital warts. In 90% of the cases genital warts are caused by low-risk types of HPV 6 and 11. However, a woman with genital warts cannot know if she has also been infected by high-risk types of HPV and must get check-ups with Pap tests or HPV tests, because prevention is the best protection against cancer.

154. What tests should you get if you develop genital warts?
In addition to a pelvic examination, you must also get a Pap test or an HPV test. Optionally, a colposcopy may also be considered, as the lower genital tract and the perianal area can be examined more thoroughly that way.

155. Can a woman with genital warts get a negative HPV test?
Yes, the HPV test is usually negative in cases of genital warts. As we mentioned above, in 90% of the cases genital warts are caused by low-risk types of HPV 6 and 11.

The HPV test is only positive when there is an infection by oncogenic types of HPV.

D) Treatment of genital warts

156. Can genital warts and HPV infection be treated?
There is no causal treatment for HPV which eradicates the virus from your body. In other words, there's no treatment for the virus itself. There are, however, treatments for the lesions which the virus might cause, i.e. for genital warts and precancerous lesions. These treatments aim only at removing or destroying the lesions.

157. What are the treatments for genital warts?
The most common treatments for genital warts are:
- Medication or substances that destroy the warts.
- Destruction of the lesions with cryotherapy, electro-cauterization or laser.
- Removal of the lesions.

158. What medications or substances are used to treat genital warts?

The substances used are podophyllotoxin, imiquimod, and trichloroacetic acid. The first two are applied by the woman herself. Trichloroacetic acid is applied by the physician and is therefore only used in a limited number of cases, where there is some relevant medical indication.

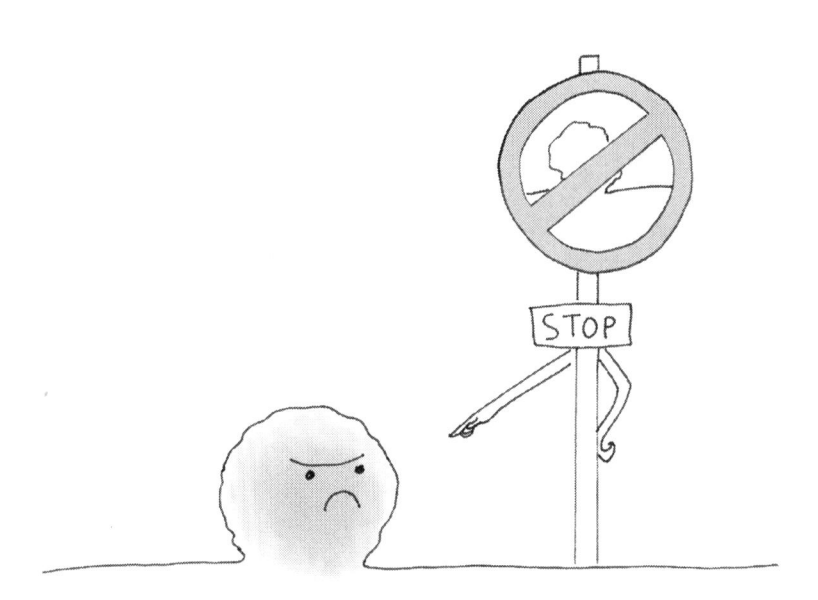

Podophyllotoxin
- Used as a solution or a cream. It is applied locally on the warts, twice a day for three days. Treatment is paused for 4 days and repeated for another 3 days. This process is usually repeated 3-4 times. The use of a

small mirror is sometimes necessary. For the solution, a cotton swab stick is usually used, while the cream is applied with the fingers. The skin of the area may become irritated.

Imiquimod cream
- This cream both destroys warts and stimulates the immune system. It causes the release of interferon and other substances locally, boosting the body's local immunity. The cream is applied locally with the fingers at night before going to bed, three times a week. After 6-10 hours, the area is rinsed to reduce irritation. The treatment may be continued for up to 16 weeks.

Ointment with sinecatechins
- This is a preparation with immune-stimulating, antioxidant, and antiviral substances (Sinecatechins/ Polyphenon E). The substances contained in the ointment come from the extract of green tea leaves (camelia sinensis plant). This ointment is applied three times a day locally, on warts of the genital organs and anal area. The treatment may last up to 12 weeks.

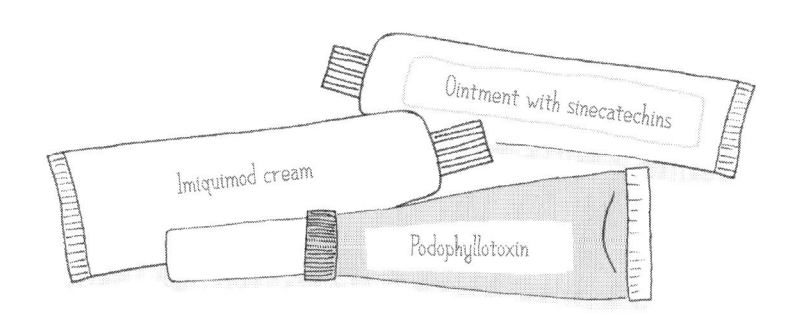

Trichloroacetic acid solution
- It is used as an 80-90% solution and is not contraindicated during pregnancy, like the other pharmaceutical treatments. A small quantity of the solution is applied by the doctor on the wart. It usually requires repeated applications once a week.

159. How are genital warts destroyed?
The usual methods are:

Destruction of genital warts with cryotherapy
- Cryotherapy is frequently used to destroy warts. The lesions are destroyed by directly freezing them, with liquid nitrogen applied as a spray or through a cryoprobe. No local anesthesia is usually given and the pain is tolerable. It is considered as a safe method during pregnancy. It is repeated every 1-2 weeks until the complete elimination of the lesions.

Electro-cauterization of the genital warts
- Electrodiathermy is applied after local anesthesia, if there is a limited number of genital warts, or after general anesthesia if the lesions are many or extensive.

Laser surgery
- Laser ablation has significant advantages, but is used more rarely compared to the other methods because it is both more costly and requires special training by the doctor.

- A significant advantage of the method is that the laser beam can be directed by the colposcope toward hard-to-reach areas, where the doctor needs more light and magnification (e.g. the vagina, anus and urethra). The method is also better compared to the others when there are a large number of warts.

FIGURE 14: Destruction of warts
1. Laser ablation
2. Cryotherapy

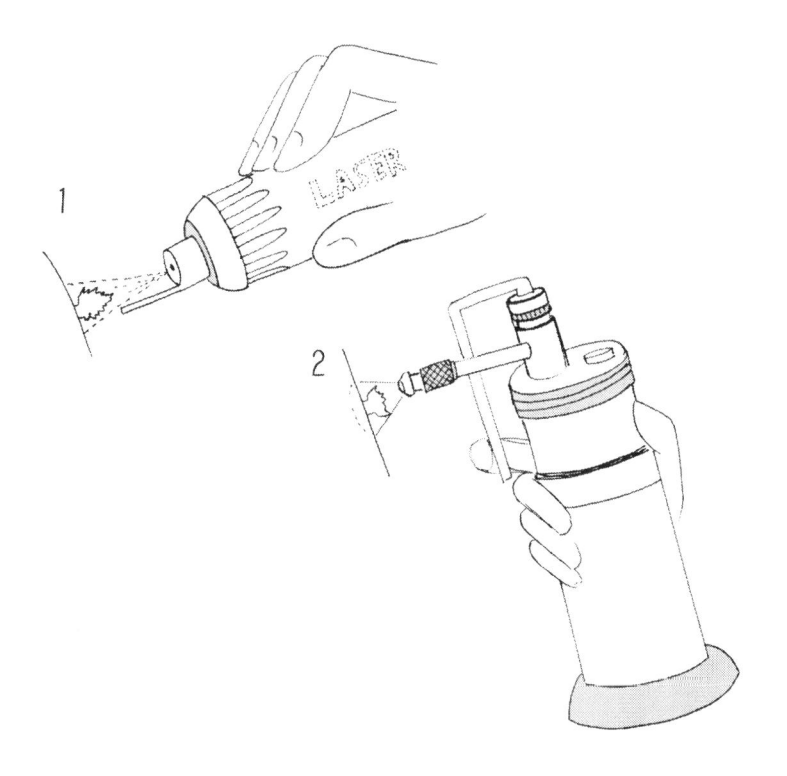

160. When and how are warts removed?

There are cases where the doctor prefers to remove a warty lesion because he would like to examine it under the microscope. This is sometimes the case with warty lesions on the cervix and vulva.

When we have small, isolated warts which do not have a broad base, it is easier to remove them under local anesthesia. Healing is fast and there will be a very good cosmetic result.

Warts may be removed with surgical scissors, scalpel or biopsy forceps.

161. Which is the best treatment for genital warts?

This will be decided by your doctor. Not all cases are the same. The doctor will reach a decision based on your history, the number of lesions, and their location. The doctor's familiarity with a specific treatment and his experience also play a role.

162. Do genital warts recur after treatment?

Unfortunately, recurrences are common. There is no treatment that ensures against the recurrence of genital warts. Recurrences are annoying and affect patients' psychology.

163. How is the recurrence of genital warts after treatment explained?

Recurrences can be explained by the fact that there is no treatment for the cause of warts. Visible lesions are destroyed, but the virus remains in the body and may create other warts. This is a matter of equilibrium. After the visible warts are removed, infectious lesions remain on the skin and mucous membranes of the genital organs, not visible to the naked eye. It is necessary for your immune system to suppress the virus for the invisible warty lesions to also disappear. It is a question of time. Sometimes it manages to do so and sometimes it doesn't, in which case we have a recurrence of warts.

It goes without saying that the entire lower genital tract and anal area must be checked each time.

You must be patient and follow your doctor's instructions.

164. How can you increase the treatment's success rates?

The good function of your immune system plays the primary role. This is why the following are recommended:
- Treating any concurrent inflammation of the lower reproductive system (e.g. vaginitis, cervicitis, etc.)
- Quit smoking
- Follow a healthy diet
- Avoid stress and get ample sleep

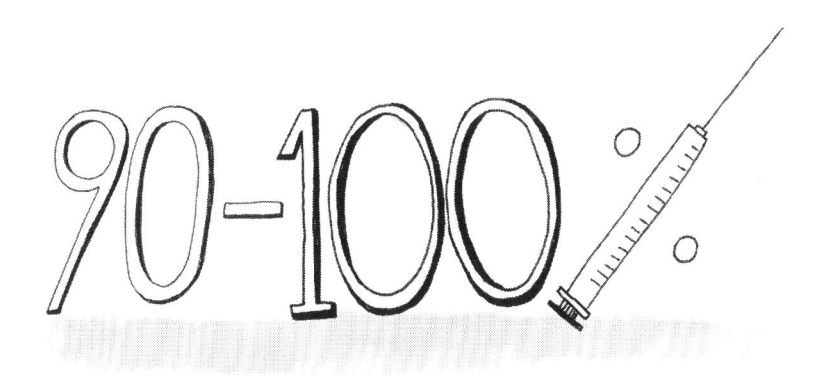

It is also recommended that you avoid shaving the genital area for a few months, because it causes small abrasions and genital warts may appear again.

E) Prevention of genital warts

165. Is there a way to prevent genital warts?

Yes, vaccination is successful in preventing genital warts at rates higher than 90%.

166. How can you protect yourself?

Genital warts are a sexually transmitted disease. Only people who have never had any sexual contact are not at risk of becoming infected.

The best prevention policy is vaccination.

The following preventive measures are also recommended:

- Restriction of the number of sexual partners
- Careful selection of your sexual partner. The more sexual partners a person has in their history, the higher the chances that they have been infected.
- Monogamous relationships are considered ideal.
- The use of a condom prevents the transmission of HPV by 70% and is recommended.
- Have regular check-ups with Pap tests and HPV tests in women, to detect in time any precancerous lesions on the cervix.

167. What should you do to avoid infecting others?

If you currently have genital warts, you must get treatment. The infection is very easily transmitted to people you have sexual intercourse with. It would be ideal not to have any contacts until the warts are treated.

However, you must also know that, for approximately 6 months after the appearance of warts, you can very easily transmit the infection to others. Therefore, it is best to use a condom during sexual intercourse.

168. Is there any point in getting vaccinated if you have ever had genital warts in the past?

The vaccine also covers other types of HPV, so you should get it. It has also been reported that, in people with warts, vaccination results in a reduction of recurrences.

Recurring respiratory papillomatosis

169. What is respiratory papillomatosis?

This is a disease where papillomas appear on the respiratory system airways (mainly the larynx and, secondarily, in the rest of the respiratory system). These papillomas may block the airways, posing a risk to the patient's life. Papillomas may appear anywhere in the respiratory system, from the nose to the lungs. However, in 95% of the cases there are lesions in the larynx. The trachea is the second most frequent area, followed by papillomas in the bronchi.

170. At what ages does it appear and how common is it?

We see it in children younger than five years old as well as adults (usually in their fourth decade). In children, the average age of diagnosis is 3.5-4 years and in adults 35-40 years.

The incidence of the disease is very low. In the USA, there are around 1,000 cases each year. A similar incidence is reported by the statistical data of Denmark.

171. What is the cause of respiratory papillomatosis?

HPV 6 and 11 are the causal factors (HPV 11 is found more frequently). HPV 16 and 18 are also found in some rare cases.

Lesions in children are attributed to their infection during childbirth. The infection of the newborn during natural childbirth is considered the most common way of transmission. It seems that a caesarean section does not protect 100%, and in some newborns HPV is also transmitted during the perinatal period. Most cases with respiratory papillomatosis are first-born children by young mothers who had a natural childbirth.

Lesions in adults are possibly due to the sexual transmission of HPV.

172. What are the symptoms?

The symptoms are:
- Hoarseness or change in voice
- Choking sensation
- Feeling a foreign object in the throat
- Coughing
- Difficulty breathing
- Wheezing when breathing

173. How is it diagnosed?

The doctor looks at the airway through a thin viewing instrument called an endoscope. During the endoscopy the doctor will examine the throat, larynx, trachea, and lower airways (laryngoscopy and bronchoscopy).

174. How is it treated?

Treatment involves the destruction of the lesions with laser, cryotherapy or microabrasion in combination with antiviral medication. Recurrences are common.

175. What is the prognosis?

The disease has remissions and flare-ups. Prognosis is worse in young children. A tracheotomy is required in many cases to ensure breathing.

In a small percentage (3-5%), the lesions may become malignant and develop into squamous cell carcinoma.

176. Is there any prevention?

Prevention is possible with the vaccine that covers HPV 6 and 11. It is considered best that both boys and girls are vaccinated before becoming sexually active. This prevents infection by the specific types of HPV and their transmission to the newborn. Vaccination before becoming sexually active also prevents against respiratory papillomatosis in adults.

CHAPTER 8
Precancerous lesions on the cervix

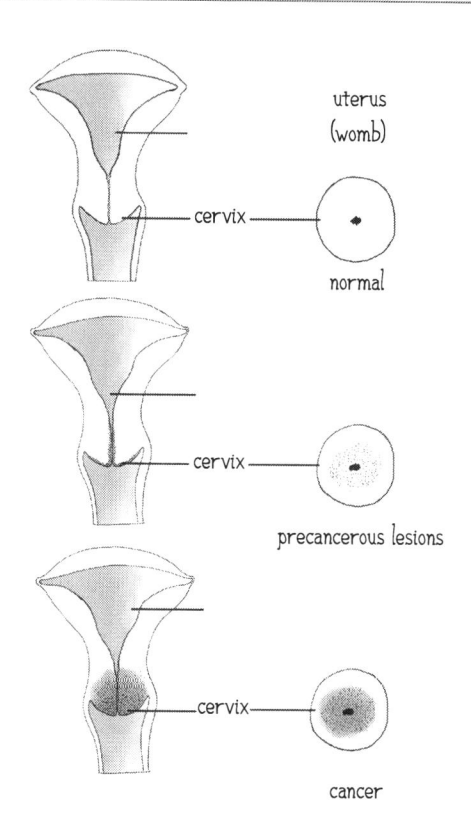

uterus (womb)

cervix

normal

cervix

precancerous lesions

cervix

cancer

From infection to precancerous lesions and cancer

177. What is the cause of cervical cancer?
The cause of cervical cancer is oncogenic (cancer-causing) or high-risk types of HPV. An oncogenic HPV type is the cause, but it is not always capable of causing cancer on its own. The human body must allow it to do so.

178. How can HPV cause cancer?
High-risk types of HPV incorporate their DNA into the human cell DNA, causing mutations. It seems that this usually happens after a chronic or recurring infection of the epithelium. See figures a-h on pages 160, 161.

DON'T FORGET:

You may have precancerous lesions for a long time and not be aware of it. They cause no symptoms! Precancerous lesions are treatable and you may prevent an invasive cancer by being careful. After treatment, however, there is a small chance of recurrence and you must continue to get check-ups.

179. What do the terms LSIL and HSIL of the cervix mean?

Infectious lesions caused by HPV are internationally referred to as LSIL (Low Grade Squamous Intraepithelial Lesions). They are otherwise referred to as low-grade lesions or condylomatous (warty) lesions.

Low-grade lesions are caused by both low-risk and high-risk HPVs (cancer-causing types).

Premalignant (precancerous) lesions caused by HPV are internationally called HSIL (High-Grade Squamous Intraepithelial Lesions). They are otherwise referred to as high-grade lesions.

Only oncogenic types of HPV (high risk – oncogenic) can cause HSIL.

The terms 'low-grade' and 'high-grade' were chosen to stress how possible it is for these lesions to grow into cancer.

Based on the above, LSILs are usually followed up, while HSIL lesions must be treated. You can find details about possible treatments in pages 166-181.

DON'T FORGET

Low-grade lesions (LSIL) have a small chance of evolving into cancer (if they have been caused by oncogenic types of HPV). On the contrary, high-grade lesions (HSIL) have a higher chance of evolving into cancer.

How can HPV cause cancer?

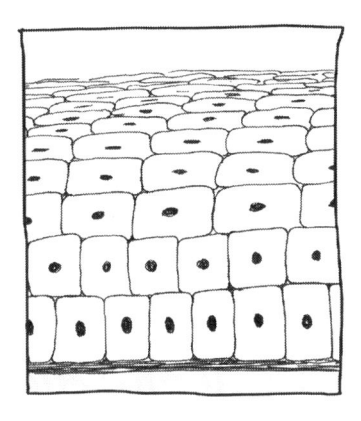

a) Normal epithelial cells

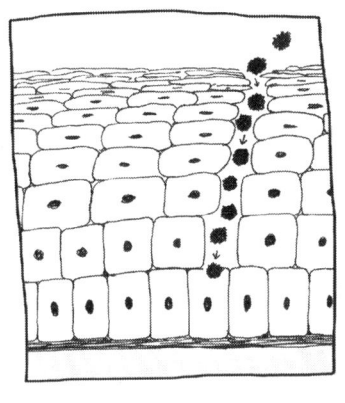

b) HPV infects the epithelium.

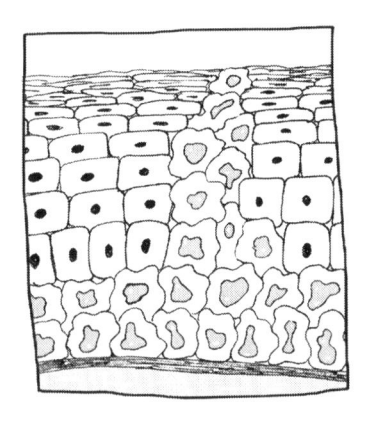

c) Lesions of the epithelial cells appear following the infection, which are usually suppressed by your body (within 6-36 months).

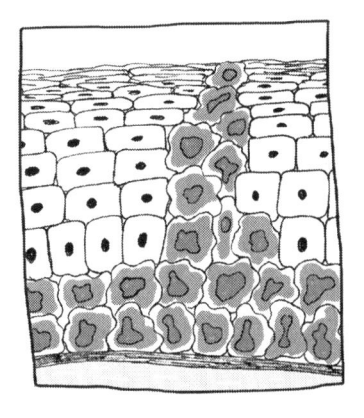

d) In a few cases the infectious lesions persist or recur.

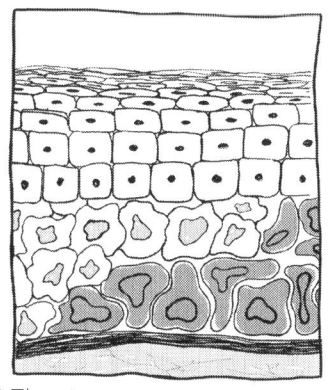

e) The virus manages to incorporate its DNA into your cells' DNA (mutation – creation of neoplastic cell).

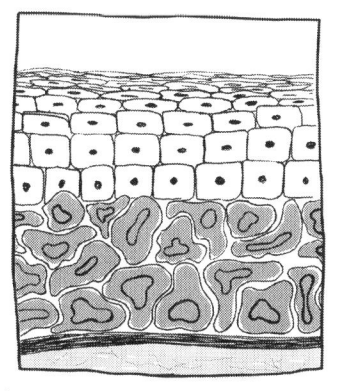

f) When there are many mutations, the multiplication of the neoplastic epithelial cells is no longer controlled by your body.

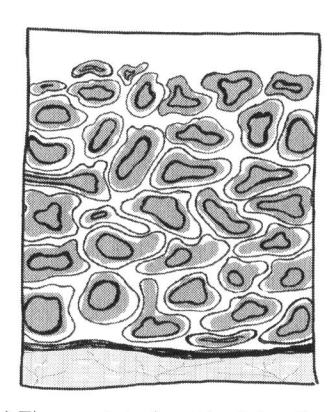

g) The mutated epithelial cells multiply at a crazy pace. They will not stay contained inside the epithelial layers but they will «break» the basal membrane and spread more deeply (invasive cancer).

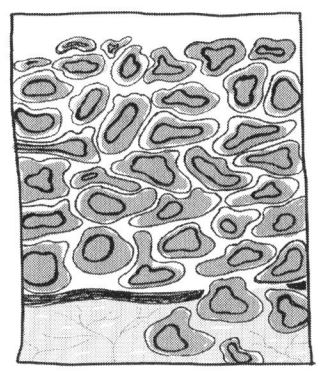

h) Under the basal membrane of the epithelium there are blood vessels. Cancer cells enter the vessels (invasion of vessels) and travel to other areas of the body (metastasis).

180. What are CIN1, CIN2, and CIN3?

CIN is the acronym for Cervical Intraepithelial Neoplasia.

CIN means that atypical cells, i.e. those which do not have the typical normal morphology are restricted to the inside of the epithelium (intraepithelial neoplasia).

Milder lesions are characterized as CIN1. In these lesions only the lower third (1/3) of the epithelium is occupied by cells with infectious atypia. CIN1 lesions are caused by both low-risk and oncogenic types of HPV.

The more severe lesions are characterized as CIN2 and, CIN3. In these lesions the lower two-thirds (2/3) or the entire thickness of the epithelium (3/3) respectively, are occupied by neoplastic cells. CIN2 and CIN3 lesions are only caused by oncogenic types of HPV.

CIN3 lesions are characterized as Carcinoma In Situ (CIS) when the entire thickness of the epithelium is completely occupied by neoplastic cells.

181. What is the prognosis for CIN1, CIN2, and CIN3/CIS?

CIN1 lesions usually subside on their own (in 80-90% of cases) within 2-3 years after the biopsies and diagnosis. This is why the term «intraepithelial neoplasia» is considered an exaggeration. It is believed that this kind of cell atypia is due to simple infection from HPV (infectious atypia). This is why CIN1 lesions are classified as LSIL (low-grade lesions).

On the contrary, CIN2 and CIN3 lesions have a significant possibility of evolving into invasive cancer in the following years. This is why they are classified as HSIL (high-grade lesions). If CIN2/3 or HSIL lesions aren't treated, there is a future risk of invasive cancer. The risk

PRECANCEROUS LESIONS ON THE CERVIX

is estimated at 30-40% of all cases, but is lower at younger ages and higher after the age of 30. The risk for carcinogenesis (development of cancer) increases with age.

CIN3 lesions have a higher risk for invasive cancer.

Especially in regard to CIN3 and CIS lesions, the lifetime risk is estimated at 60-80%. Women older than 30, with CIN3/CIS lesions covering a large part of the cervical surface, are at the highest risk.

182. Which terms are used internationally for precancerous lesions on the cervix?

The terms HSIL, CIN2, CIN3, CIS, and AIS are used internationally to describe premalignant cervical lesions.

You can see these acronyms in the Pap test results or the histological report of a cervical biopsy.

Since certain terms are synonymous, their synonyms are referred to in summary in Table 5 (p. 164), together with the meaning of each term.

TABLE 5
The names of premalignant cervical lesions and their meaning

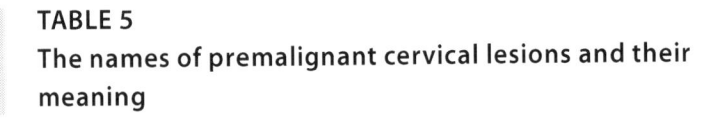

NAME OF LESIONS	SYNONYM	MEANING
HSIL	CIN2/CIN3	High-Grade Squamous Intraepithelial Lesions.
CIN2	HSIL	Squamous Cell Lesions occupying 2/3 of the epithelial thickness.
CIN3/CIS	HSIL	Squamous Cell Lesions occupying 3/3 of the epithelial thickness. Significant risk of invasive squamous cell cancer.
AIS		Serious premalignant lesion on the glandular epithelium. Significant risk of adenocarcinoma.

What does the diagnosis involve?

183. Are cervical precancerous lesions visible during a gynecological examination? How are they discovered?

Precancerous lesions on the cervix are not visible to the naked eye. They are usually microscopic lesions inside the epithelium. They cannot be spotted by your doctor during a typical gynecological examination.

This is why your doctor will combine the gynecological examination with a Pap test or an HPV test. If there are any anomalous findings in these tests, the next step is usually a colposcopy and biopsy.

Don't wait to see symptoms to go to your doctor. Premalignant lesions cause no symptom.

184. Why should lesions be found when they are still invisible to the naked eye examination?

Because cancer is prevented only in the phase when the cancer cells are restricted to the epithelium and have not spread more deeply.

When we refer to precancerous lesions, we mean those inside the epithelium (intraepithelial lesions), which are invisible to the naked eye.

Under the epithelium, there are blood vessels and lymphatic vessels. If the cancer cells spread under the epithelium, they enter the vessels and travel to other areas of the body where they "take residence". In this case, we are talking about a metastasis.

185. What are the necessary tests and in what order should they be performed?

Usually, a Pap test showing suspect cells or a positive HPV test are followed by a colposcopy.

The doctor performing the colposcopy assesses whether to perform biopsies or remove a larger part of tissue (cone biopsy).

In order to reach a definite diagnosis, some or all of the following tests may be required:
- Pap test
- HPV test
- Colposcopy
- Histologic examination of biopsies or part of the cervix
- Histologic examination of a tissue sample from the cervical canal.

Treatment of cervical precancerous lesions

186. What is the purpose of the treatment?

The purpose of the treatment is to destroy or remove not only the precancerous lesions but the entire transformation zone.

The reason is simple. The transformation zone is the cervical area where HPV causes cancer. Its removal is therefore considered imperative.

Frequently, after the transformation zone is removed and the tissue is examined under the microscope, the lesions that are found are more serious than what the Pap test or the colposcopic biopsies had showed.

187. What treatments are there available?

We distinguish between removal methods and destruction methods:

Excisional (removal) methods:
- LEEP
- Laser conization
- Cold knife conization

Ablative (destruction) methods
- Laser
- Cryotherapy

188. How is the most appropriate method selected?

The best method is chosen by the doctor, based on the patient's best interest. The parameters that help him decide correctly are the severity of the lesions, the patient's age and the risk for underlying cancer, and the patient's future fertility.

Excisional methods are selected if the removed tissue must be examined because we suspect that there may be more serious underlying lesions. Among removal methods, LEEP is used more frequently (see a detailed description in pages 171-175).

189. What are the criteria used to choose the correct treatment for the lesions?

The risk for invasive cancer is assessed. We take into consideration the specific patient's history and the findings from her tests.

LSIL/CIN1 lesions have a relatively low risk. But the risk changes, depending on whether they were caused by HPV16, HPV18 or other types of HPV.

If we are certain of the diagnosis, we follow up these cases closely. Some of them will present HSIL/CIN2, CIN3 in the near or more distant future, in which case they must be treated.

If we are uncertain of the diagnosis, especially in older patients, and we are afraid of underlying HSIL/CIN2 or CIN3 lesions, it is preferable that we treat them immediately.

HSIL/CIN2, and CIN3 lesions have a significant risk of invasive cancer in the future.

Not all cases with this diagnosis are the same. Let's take two extreme examples of women with the same diagnosis (HSIL/CIN2, 3), who could follow a different treatment.

In the first case, it is a 20-year-old young woman with HSIL diagnosis in the Pap test. She had a colposcopy, and small lesions were found. The doctor took biopsies and the histological diagnosis is CIN2.

In the second case it is a 38-year-old woman, also with an HSIL diagnosis from the Pap test. The colposcopy, however, found extensive lesions occupying the whole transformation zone on her cervix and the biopsies showed CIN2 and CIN3.

What is of interest to us is firstly the risk of missing an underlying invasive cancer, and second, the risk of invasive cancer appearing in the immediate future.

In a 20-year old young woman, the risk of underlying invasive cancer is nearly non-existent. In a 38-year-old woman, the risk is significant. In the young woman's case, the risk of appearance of invasive cancer in the immediate future is low, and she could be closely followed up, without immediate treatment at this time. In the 38-year-old woman's case, the risk is very high, and she must undergo treatment immediately.

190. What happens if HSIL or CIN2/3 lesions are discovered during pregnancy?

If we are certain about the diagnosis and we don't have any suspicion of underlying cancer, we must follow up the lesions, and they must be treated after the pregnancy.

Description of procedures

191. What is the logic behind these procedures?

Precancerous lesions are usually located in the transformation zone. The transformation zone is the cervical area where oncogenic types of HPV cause squamous cell cancer. Glandular cell cancer is rarer and affects the glandular epithelium that covers the cervical canal on the inside (see Figure 8, p. 102).

These procedures do not eradicate HPV virus from the woman's body.

The procedures treat precancerous lesions and remove or destroy the transformation zone, which is the fertile ground on which the oncogenic virus will cause new lesions. This significantly reduces the probability of a recurrence of premalignant lesions and cancer.

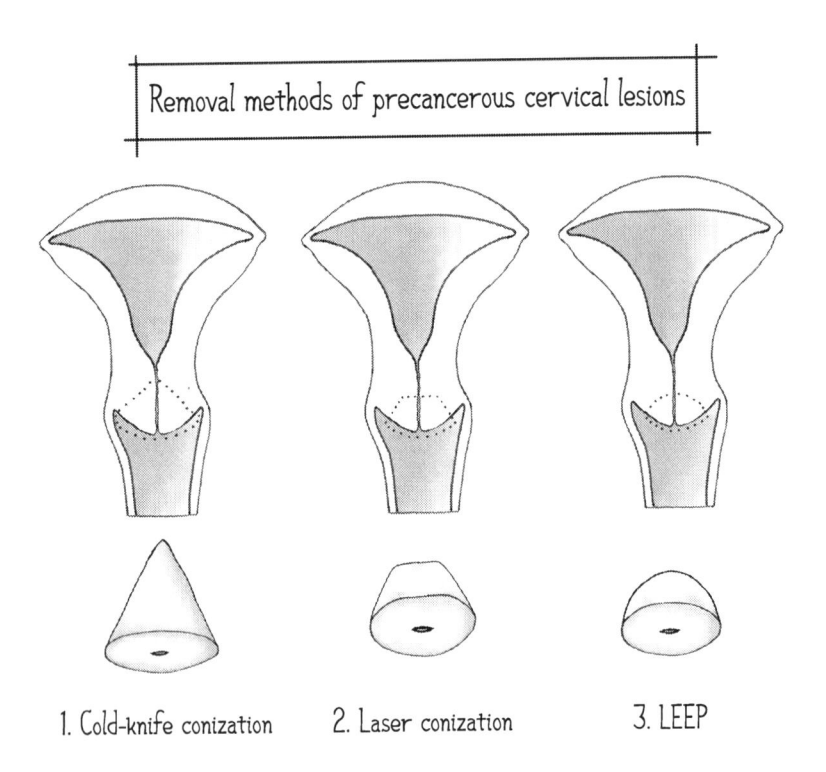

Removal methods of precancerous cervical lesions

1. Cold-knife conization   2. Laser conization   3. LEEP

192. What should the patient do to prepare before the procedure?

- The possibility of pregnancy must be excluded.
- The patient is examined for any co-existing inflammation. If inflammation (e.g. from chlamydia, etc.) is discovered, she must be treated before the procedure.
- The procedure is scheduled immediately after the end of her menstruation.
- Before the procedure, the patient is informed in detail about the benefits and risks and possible complications and signs a consent form.

Procedures for the removal of the transformation zone

A) LEEP

193. What does it mean?

LEEP are the initials for Loop Electrosurgical Excision Procedure.

This procedure is also referred to as LLETZ (Large Loop Excision of the Transformation Zone). It is the excision of the transformation zone tissue by using an electrical loop.

The Loop is made of a thin wire, with a high-frequency current running through it. Thanks to the current running through it, the wire loop cuts through the tissue and removes it.

194. Does the LEEP procedure require general anesthesia?

No general anesthesia is required normally, because the procedure is usually well-tolerated with local anesthesia.

General anesthesia is administered when there are anatomical particularities (e.g. a displaced cervix), and access to the surgical field is difficult. Also, in cases where the lesions cover a large area and extend to the vaginal vaults or when curettage is also necessary.

195. How is the procedure performed?

- The patient lies in the gynecological examination position.
- The doctor inserts the speculum into the vagina (like when performing a Pap test) and opens the vaginal walls to have visual access to the surgical field. He cleans the vagina with normal saline and antiseptic solution.

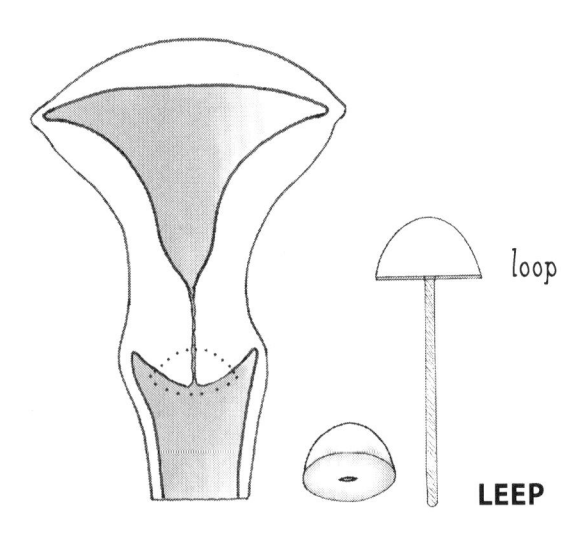

PRECANCEROUS LESIONS ON THE CERVIX 173

- The doctor then inspects the cervix through the colposcope, after using an acetic acid solution, and if necessary, an iodine solution called 'lugol'. He identifies the lesion areas and the transformation zone, i.e. the part of the tissue that must be removed.
- Local anesthesia is performed on the cervix, using a thin dental needle.
- The loop size is chosen, depending on the anatomical position of the lesions and the size of the transformation zone.
- The loop is connected with the electrodiathermy machine and the current is activated by the doctor as the loop moves, dissects and removes the tissue.
- The tissue with the lesions is usually removed in one go, i.e. by passing the loop once over it. However, in patients with extensive lesions, a second passage of the loop may be required.
- After the tissue is removed, the bleeding areas are identified and cauterized with electrodiathermy.
  The procedure does not require hospitalization of the patient. Hospitalization is required only in a few high-risk cases, when the doctor deems it necessary.

196. What are the complications and risks of a LEEP procedure?

Complications after a LEEP procedure are not frequent (they occur in <10% of cases). According to the informational leaflet of the American Society for Colposcopy and Cervical Pathology (ASCCP), which is given to patients before a procedure, the following complications are possible:
- Heavy bleeding
- Bleeding with clots

- Severe abdominal pain described as a cramp
- Fever
- Vaginal odorous discharge - Post-op inflammation
- Occasional cutting or burning of normal tissue
- Imperfect removal of infected tissue
- Stenosis of cervical opening after the procedure

The ASCCP patient information leaflet also mentions that the patient must inform the doctor if, after leaving the hospital, she has any of the following:
- Bleeding (blood quantity greater than a period or clots)
- Fever
- Yellow vaginal pus-like discharge, or odorous discharge.

If she can't find her doctor, the patient must go to the ER.

197. Post-operative instructions

After the procedure, a painkiller is recommended. To prevent any post-operative bleeding or inflammation, you must do the following for 4 weeks:
- Don't lift weights heavier than 5-6 kg.
- No sexual contact.
- Do not insert anything into your vagina (tampons, vaginal douche, fingers, vibrators, etc).

198. What are the future risks after a LEEP procedure?

Apart from the small chance of stenosis of the cervical opening, it has been observed that the removal of large parts of the cervix contributes to an increase in the frequency of premature labor in future pregnancies.

The increase is small if the procedure is performed once and the volume of the removed tissue does not exceed 25% of the total volume of the cervix. It increases, however, in those cases where large parts are removed or a second LEEP is done.

B) COLD-KNIFE CONIZATION

199. What is it?

It is the excision of a cone-shaped part of the cervix with a surgical scalpel.

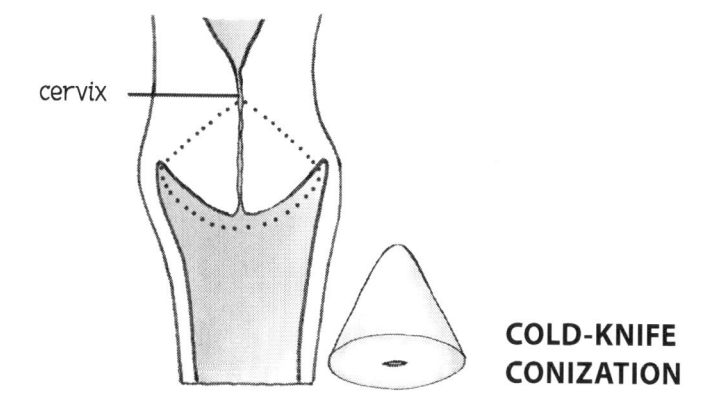

COLD-KNIFE CONIZATION

200. When is it performed?

Cold-knife conization is very limited nowadays due to the wide-spread use of the LEEP procedure.

A cold-knife conization is performed:
- When there is suspicion of adenocarcinoma.
- In cases of high-risk lesions that extend high into the cervical canal.
- If smears of the cervical canal reveal serious lesions that were not detected by the colposcopy.

201. How is the procedure performed?

The patient is admitted to the hospital. The procedure is done under general anesthesia. The cervix is cut with a scalpel and a cone-shaped part is removed, including the transformation zone and part of the cervical canal. Hemostasis is performed, and sutures are placed for the anatomical restoration of the trauma.

202. What are the procedure's risks?

The risks from a conization are:
- Bleeding
- Inflammation
- Trauma to adjacent tissues and the vagina
- Fertility problems
- Stenosis of the cervical canal
- Increased chances of premature birth in future pregnancies

C) LASER CONIZATION

203. What is it and what are its advantages?

A focused laser beam is used in laser conization instead of a scalpel.

The laser beam (carbon dioxide) dissects the cervical tissue, just like the scalpel. But it has the advantage that at the same time small vessels are cauterized and the bleeding is reduced.

The beam is directed onto the tissue by a special control pad attached to the colposcope. The doctor views the surgical field through the colposcope. A significant advantage of this method is that it can be done under local anesthesia.

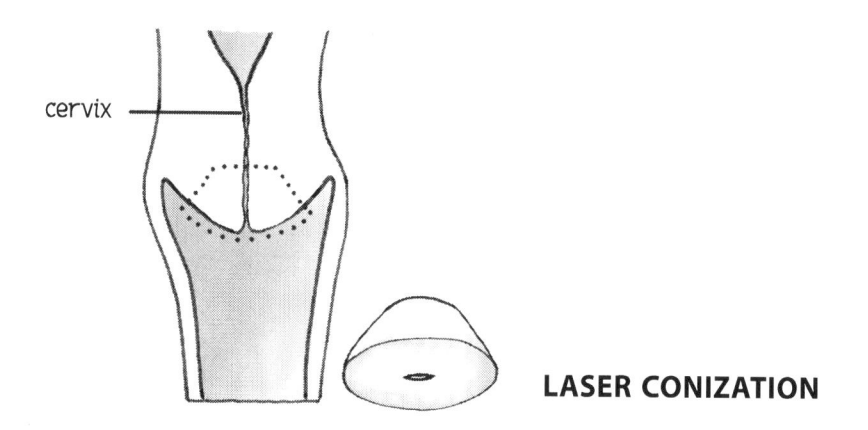

LASER CONIZATION

204. In which cases is it preferred?

First of all, the hospital must have the laser device available (which is very expensive). This procedure also requires training and experience of the doctor that will perform it.

With this technique, the doctor may remove with precision the part of the tissue with the lesions and modify the shape of the excision. For example, he may remove a part of the cervix that is not cone-shaped but cylindrical (this is done when the transformation zone extends high up into the cervical canal).

205. What are its complications?

The complications are the same as in the LEEP procedure.

Procedures that destroy the transformation zone

The procedures that destroy the transformation zone are:
- laser ablation and
- cryosurgery.

Due to the destruction of the tissue during the procedure, there can be no histologic examination. Therefore none of these techniques are used when there is even the smallest possibility of a starting squamous or glandular cell carcinoma hiding inside the tissue to be destroyed.

D) LASER ABLATION OF THE TRANSFORMATION ZONE

206. What is it and how is it done?
The transformation zone and the lesions are destroyed with a carbon dioxide laser that is aimed through the colposcope.

Local anesthesia is used in the procedure, which is well-tolerated. The doctor ablates the transformation zone tissues by moving the laser beam over the cervical tissue. The tissue must be ablated to a depth of 6-8 mm in order to also destroy the epithelium inside the gland crypts.

207. What are the advantages and disadvantages of the method?
It has many advantages.
- The procedure is done under local anesthesia.
- Only the precise area is ablated. This minimizes the risk for premature labor in the future.
- If the technique is correct, healing is excellent.
- There is no significant increase in the frequency of premature labor in patients that have had this procedure, compared to the rest of the population.

The disadvantages are:
- There is no possibility of a histologic examination, since the tissue is destroyed.
- It is an expensive method due to the cost of the equipment and requires the doctor's special training.

E) CRYOTHERAPY

208. How is it done?
Cryotherapy or cryosurgery in general, is the procedure of freezing tissue to kill and remove abnormal tissues or growths (warts, etc.) Cryotherapy for treating CIN was used often in the past, but is used less and less these days.

It is a simple procedure. With the help of a special device, the transformation zone area is frozen to minus 68-85 degrees Celsius for 3 minutes. The area is then left to defrost for 5 minutes and the freezing procedure is repeated for 3 more minutes.

After this procedure, the tissue dies and drops off. The patient is warned that over the next days she will have increased vaginal discharge. The area of cryotherapy is covered by new epithelium within 6 weeks.

209. What are the advantages and disadvantages of the method?
It has the following advantages:
- It is cheap and does not require a particularly specialized doctor.
- It is performed without any anesthesia. A painkiller about an hour before the procedure is usually sufficient.
- The volume of cervical tissue that is destroyed is not significant (the risk for premature labor does not increase).

There are, however, significant disadvantages:
- It is not always certain that the tissue will be destroyed deep enough. If the affected tissue is not destroyed and gland crypts remain under the trauma, there is future risk, which is frequently hard to detect with a simple Pap test.
- Stenosis of the cervical opening is much more frequent after cryotherapy (compared to other methods), and occurs in 3-5% of the cases.

Post-operative follow-up and recurrences

210. Is follow-up necessary after the lesions are treated?

Patients are always informed about the need for follow-up after the treatment. They are told, in particular, that no treatment eradicates HPV, and therefore the possibility for recurrence of the lesions may be small, but it does exist (it is 2%-3%).

Patients with an HSIL history must be checked in their entire lower genital tract.

After HSIL treatment, follow-up is every six months for the two first years. A greater frequency of recurrences has been observed during this period. After two years, and if no problems have been observed, check-ups are necessary once a year. It is stressed, however, to patients that they must comply with the time frames.

211. Will you be transmitting the HPV infection after treatment?

This depends on two things. First, on how successful the treatment was, and whether all visible lesions have been eliminated. Ssecond, on the state of your immune system and its capability of suppressing the HPV that remains after the lesions are destroyed. Usually, after the lesions are removed, a 6-12 month period passes until the HPV is suppressed by the immune system, and infectiousness is drastically reduced.

212. If you get treatment and the HPV lesions are gone, is there a risk of becoming reinfected by your partner?

Even if the visible HPV lesions are removed or destroyed, sometimes the virus remains in the lower genital tract area, in latent form. This is why recurrences are possible, regardless of whether we come in contact again with the person that transmitted the virus to us.

Lesions usually reappear because the immune system is not yet capable of suppressing the virus. It is all a matter of balance between the viral action of HPV (which depends on the type of the virus) and the body's immune system (cellular defenses against HPVs). In the case of a recent infection, since we do not know if our immune system has reached a satisfactory performance, we recommend the use of a condom for a few months. Also, after treatment, the use of a condom for six months has been proven beneficial, obviously because it stops the building of a new viral load.

CHAPTER 9

Precancerous lesions caused by HPV in the vagina, vulva, and anus

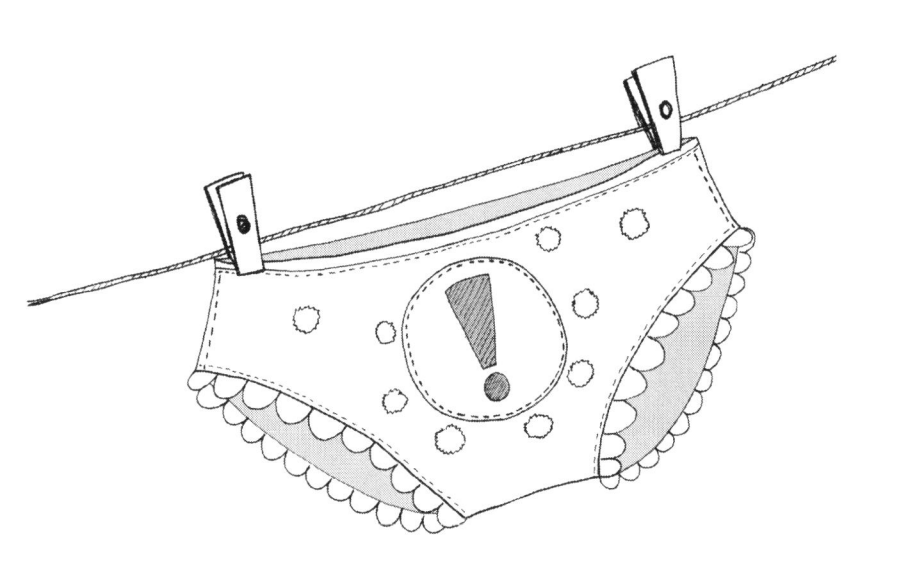

Vaginal precancerous lesions (VaIN)

213. What are VaINs?

VaINs are lesions with abnormal cells inside the vaginal epithelium. VaIN are the initials of the words Vaginal Intraepithelial Neoplasia.

Vaginal lesions are distinguished into:
- low-grade (LSIL/VaIN1) and
- high-grade (HSIL/VaIN2,3)

The classification is similar to the lesions on the cervical squamous epithelium.

The term low-grade signifies the good behavior of the lesions of this group, which are usually simple condylomatous (warty) infections and subside on their own.

The term high-grade signifies the possibility of these lesions evolving into invasive vaginal cancer.

214. How are they diagnosed?

Most of the VaIN lesions are discovered during the colposcopy which follows an abnormal Pap test.

The doctor detects the lesions on the vagina after first applying an acetic acid solution and then the lugol iodine solution. The next step is to take biopsies in order to ascertain the severity of the lesions with a histologic examination.

215. Which lesions require treatment?

Low-grade lesions (LSIL/VaIN1) usually subside without any treatment.

In young women, VaIN2 lesions should be monitored for a certain period because a significant percentage of them subside automatically.

Even though the physical history of carcinogenesis in the vagina has not been fully explained, it is internationally accepted that high-grade lesions (HSIL/VaIN2, 3), and in particular VaIN3, must be treated.

216. How are high-grade lesions (HSIL/VaIN2, 3) treated?

There are two methods for treating the lesions:
- Laser ablation of the lesions
- Excision of the lesions

Ablation is performed when there is no suspicion that invasive carcinoma on the vaginal wall may have been missed. When there is any suspicion of invasive cancer, the removal of the lesions is preferred.

217. Can vaginal precancerous lesions appear in women who have had their uterus removed?

Women with a history of high-grade cervical lesions or cervical cancer have a risk of precancerous vaginal lesions and vaginal cancer after a hysterectomy.

Follow-up is recommended for these women.

218. What is the effect of smoking on VaIN lesions?

Smoking is considered to have an exacerbating role and quitting is recommended. Smoking is believed to increase the possibility of carcinogenesis or recurrence of the lesions after treatment.

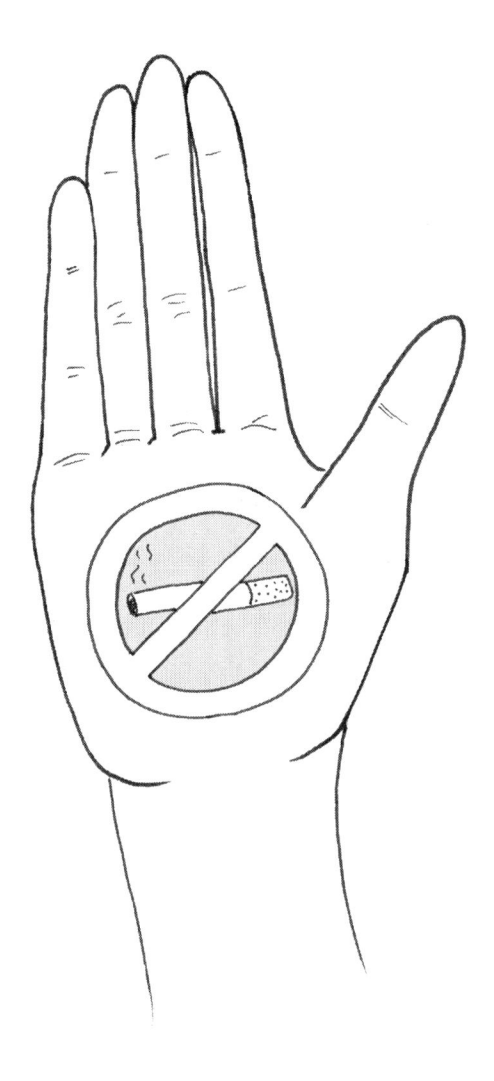

HPV-related precancerous lesions of the vulva (VIN)

219. What does VIN mean?

The term VIN refers to precancerous lesions of the vulva (Vulvar Intraepithelial Neoplasia).

A percentage of vulvar cancers (approximately 40%) is causally related to oncogenic types of HPV. These precancerous lesions that precede cancer are referred to as "HPV-related VIN lesions."

HPV 16 is the most common causal factor.

220. How are HPV-related VIN lesions classified?

In the past, they used to be classified as VIN 1, 2, 3. The classification system has changed since 2004, however, and the term VIN today describes only high-grade lesions (VIN2, 3).

Low-grade lesions are referred to as simple condylomatous (wart-like) lesions.

221. Are HPV-related VIN lesions visible?

Most of these lesions are visible to a naked eye examination. Their color varies. They are usually gray or white. Sometimes, however, they are shades of red or brown.

HPV-related VIN lesions cause no symptoms. Itching is reported in a few cases. Quite often, they are discovered accidentally by the patient or the doctor. Patients frequently report a history of genital warts or a CIN history.

222. How are the lesions diagnosed?

The vulvar area is examined under magnification (optionally with the colposcope), as the entire lower genital tract and anal area should be examined.

Diagnosis always requires a biopsy and histological examination.

223. How are HPV-related VIN lesions treated?

As mentioned above, only high-grade lesions (VIN 2, 3) are considered VIN lesions. Treatment is recommended for these lesions.

No treatment is recommended for subclinical condylomatous lesions, which used to be referred to as VIN1.

224. What does treatment entail and what are the criteria?

The following treatments are currently recommended:
- Surgical removal of lesions: Surgical removal is necessary even when there is the slightest suspicion of an invasive vulvar carcinoma. It is also required in cases where the VIN lesions are in vulvar areas covered with hair, because the affected epithelium in these areas goes down deep around the hair follicles, and cannot be destroyed with a surface laser.
- Ablation of lesions with carbon dioxide laser: This method is considered the best for the destruction of the lesions. It is implemented by your doctor only in vulvar areas with no hair (for the reason mentioned above). Healing is very good, as is the cosmetic result.

- Imiquimod cream: It was first used as an adjunct treatment to the previous treatments in order to decrease recurrences. It is also administered in selected cases as a first-line treatment (small lesions, that have recently appeared in young women), with close follow-up.

225. Do the lesions recur after treatment? Is follow-up necessary?

Recurrences of the lesions after treatment are very common. Therefore, close follow-up is required.

Precancerous lesions of the anal canal (AIN) and the perianal area (PaIN)

226. What are AIN lesions?

Precancerous lesions that precede the appearance of cancer in the anal canal have been clearly described.

In the anal canal, at the sphincter level, we find metaplastic epithelium (like in the cervix). Intraepithelial lesions caused by HPV in the area are called AIN (Anal Intraepithelial Neoplasia).

It is believed that AIN lesions behave like the corresponding CIN lesions in the cervix (they both start in metaplastic type squamous epithelium).

227. How are AIN lesions classified?

The classification of AIN lesions is similar to that of cervical CIN lesions.

If the atypical cells cover the entire thickness of the epithelium, the lesions are classified as AIN3. In those cases where they cover the two lower thirds, they are called AIN2. When they only cover the lower third of the epithelium, they are called AIN1.

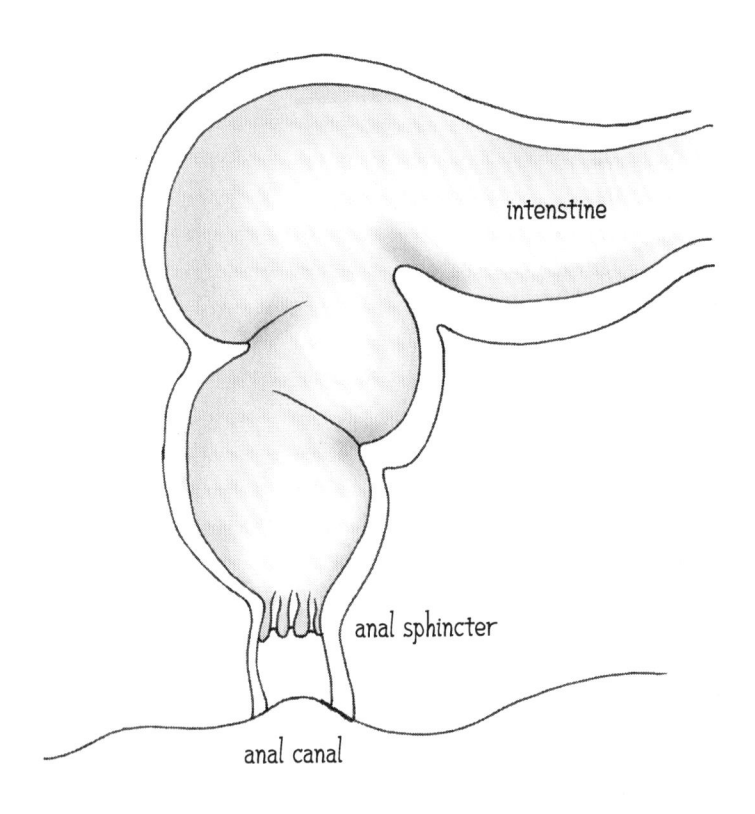

intenstine

anal sphincter

anal canal

228. What is the prognosis for AIN lesions?

The physical history of carcinogenesis in the anal canal has not been fully clarified, like it has for the cervix. However, several studies have been published in the past ten years, which lead to similar conclusions as regards the potential of the lesions for carcinogenesis.

AIN1 lesions are considered mild infectious lesions. They are also called low-grade and are referred to with the international term LSIL.

AIN2 and AIN3 lesions are classified as "high-grade" or HSIL and are considered precancerous.

229. What are PaIN lesions and how can they be classified?

PaIN (Peri-Anal Intraepithelial Neoplasia): Intraepithelial Neoplasia of the skin epithelium in the perianal area.

The behavior of PaIN lesions is similar to that of VIN lesions (in the vulva).

230. Who is at risk for AIN and PaIN?

The following are considered high-risk groups for AIN:
- People who engage in anal sex are at risk for AIN and PaIN
- The risk appears to increase in older ages and smokers
- People with a history of genital warts in the anus
- People with chronic immunosuppression due to HIV infection (AIDS)
- People under chronic pharmaceutical immunosuppression (patients with transplanted organs, chronic users of cortisone, etc.)
- Women with a history of precancerous lesions in the lower reproductive system

231. What preventive measures are recommended?
- Vaccination
- Screening of population groups that are considered high-risk in order to detect any lesions
- Safe sex with use of a condom, careful selection of sexual partners, restriction of the number of sexual partners.
- Quitting smoking
- A healthy lifestyle

232. Are there symptoms from the AIN/PaIN lesions?
There are usually no symptoms. In isolated cases, patients report itching or unusual anal discharge.

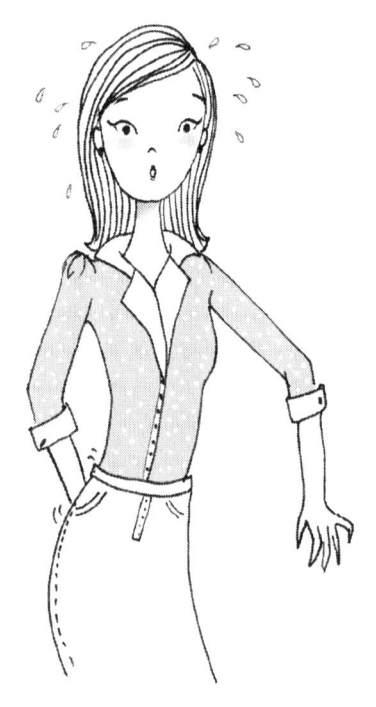

233. How are the lesions diagnosed?
It is considered useful for high-risk groups to have check-ups after a certain age. There are no clear instructions yet, but considering that anal cancer usually appears after the age of 50, it would be reasonable to start getting check-ups before that.

The Pap test (collecting cells from the anal canal) is already used as a preventive check-up method. Its reliability is not very high (as it is in the cervix) and it is believed that in the future it will be combined with molecular techniques.

The examination of the mucosa of the anal canal and the skin of the perianal area with the colposcope, called High-Resolution Anoscopy, is considered very reliable for finding precancerous AIN and PaIN lesions. If lesions are discovered, biopsies are taken.

A digital rectal examination must always be performed to exclude a palpable tumor.

234. How are AIN/PaIN lesions treated?

PaIN lesions are treated the same way as VIN lesions.

AIN lesions require the doctor's specialization in the field, because their treatment is not always easy and there are frequent complications.

235. Which AIN lesions require treatment?

It is recommended that only HSIL lesions are treated, and in particular AIN3 lesions. Some cases with AIN2 lesions can be followed up with biopsies over a certain period.

236. How are high-grade lesions (HSIL/AIN2, 3) treated?

Many methods have been tried.

Among non-surgical methods, it appears that the imiquimod cream has relatively good results.

Among surgical techniques, laser ablation of the epithelium or cauterisation are preferred when there is no suspicion of underlying invasive cancer.

In serious lesions, where the possibility of invasive cancer cannot be excluded, the lesions are removed with a scalpel, and an effort is made to anatomically restore the area. This is easier in the case of lesions that do not spread out more than 1/3 of the perimeter of the anal canal.

237. Do AIN and PaIN lesions recur after treatment? Is follow-up necessary?

Both PaIN and AIN lesions frequently recur after treatment and require regular follow-up.

Quitting smoking is also recommended. Smoking is an exacerbating factor for carcinogenesis from HPV in the anus, as well as in the lower genital tract in general.

238. How frequent are HSIL/AIN2, 3 lesions in the general population?

The incidence of HSIL/AIN2, 3 lesions is currently considered to be less than 1% in the general population. There are, however, indications that this percentage will increase in the future due to the epidemic of infections by HPV.

239. Are women with high-grade lesions (HSIL) in an organ at an increased risk for similar lesions in other organs?

The risk is clearly higher than the rest of the population and the recommendation is to monitor the entire lower genital tract and the anal area.

For example, women with a CIN3 history have increased risk for carcinogenesis from HPV in other areas. More specifically:
- Seven times higher risk for vaginal cancer
- Two times higher risk for vulvar cancer
- Five times higher risk for anal cancer

CHAPTER 10

Cancers caused by genital types of HPV

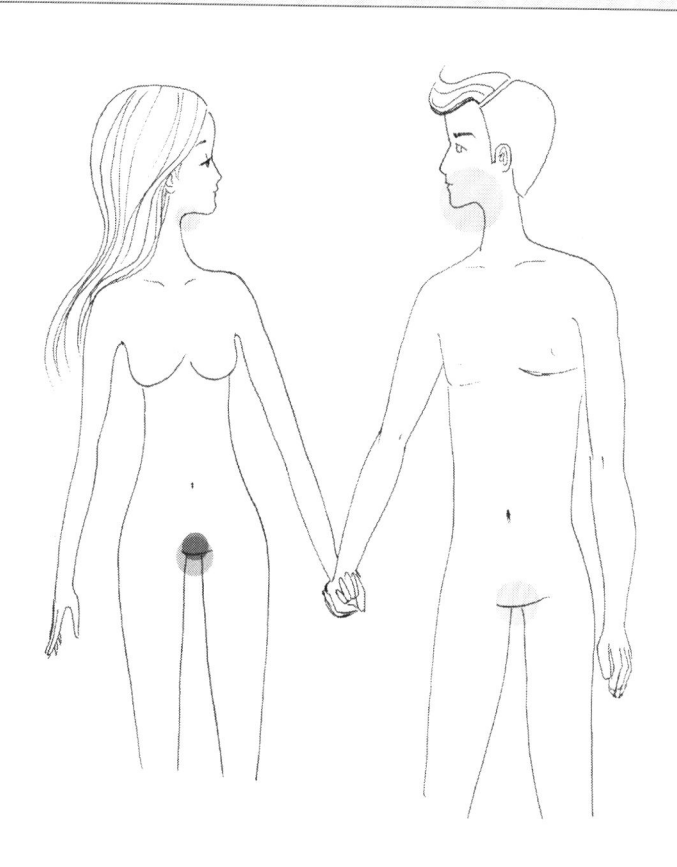

240. What is cancer?

Cancer is a genetic disease – that is, it is caused by changes in genes that control the way our cells function, especially how they grow and divide.

Our body consists of billions of cells. Our cells have a life cycle. Normally, human cells grow and divide to form new cells as the body needs them. When cells grow old or become damaged, they die, and new cells take their place.

When we are children, our cells multiply at a faster pace as our body grows. If we get injured, our cells multiply faster in the injured area and replace the lost tissue. As we get older, new cells usually just replace the cells that have aged and died.

There is a constant renewal of the cells in our body, which is well-controlled by the special mechanisms we have available. In question 11 of the first chapter (p. 57) we described how cells in our epithelium are renewed. If control is lost during any phase, and some cells start multiplying uncontrollably, tumors are formed (carcinogenesis).

The carcinogenesis process is very different than the normal cell multiplication process. The orderly process described above breaks down.

The main role is held by the DNA in each cell. If our DNA is damaged for some reason, this is called a mutation, and results in mutated daughter cells that do not function normally. Mutated (cancer) cells, apart from not functioning normally, also multiply uncontrollably without ever stopping, don't die, and form tumors.

Cancerous tumors can spread into, or invade, nearby tissues. In addition, as these tumors grow, some cancer cells can break off and travel to distant places of the body through the blood or the lymph system and form new tumors far from the original tumor (metastases).

The reasons for the appearance of mutated cells and cancer are many, such as:
- Heredity
- Radiation
- Chemical carcinogens
- Infectious factors

As we explained in the first chapter (question 19, pp. 64, 65), the DNA of oncogenic types of HPV, after chronic infection of the epithelium, may cause mutations in our cells with a possibility of carcinogenesis.

241. In which organs do genital types of HPV cause cancer?

Based on the scientific data we have available, high-risk genital types of HPV may cause cancer in the following organs:
- Uterine cervix
- Vagina
- Vulva
- Anus (in women and men)
- Head and neck (in women and men)
- Penis

242. Does HPV cause all the cancers in the above organs?

According to the latest scientific data, oncogenic types of HPV are considered a causal factor for:
- nearly all cervical cancers
- >90% of anal cancers

- 40% of vulvar cancers
- 60% of vaginal cancers
- 40-50% of penile cancers
- 25-35% of head and neck cancers

243. Other than an oncogenic type of HPV, are there other factors that lead to carcinogenesis?

Generally speaking, a risk factor for carcinogenesis in an organ can be anything that increases your risk for cancer.

Different cancers have different risk factors. Some of these factors (e.g. smoking) are something you can change (quit smoking). Other factors, such as age or family history, cannot change.

If you have a risk factor, this does not mean that you will get cancer, just that your chances are higher. Many people have multiple risk factors and never develop cancer.

In this case we are referring to cancers attributed to oncogenic types of HPV.

Once HPV enters an epithelial cell, the virus begins to make the proteins it encodes. Two of the proteins made by high-risk HPVs (E6 and E7) interfere with cell functions that normally prevent excessive growth, helping the mutated cancer cell to grow in an uncontrolled manner and avoid cell death.

As has been proven, besides the causal factor (HPV), there are other parameters that also play a role.

The immune system

The study of carcinogenesis in the cervix has shown that the cell infection caused by a high-risk type of HPV can lead to the appearance of cells with mutated DNA.

Our immune system's mechanisms suppress infections. People whose immune system is not functioning properly (e.g. AIDS patients) have higher chances of carcinogenesis from HPV.

Another group of patients with a suppressed immune system are those who are taking immunosuppressant drugs (cortisone, cyclosporine, etc.) because they have a chronic condition or have had an organ transplant.

History of other cancers or precancerous lesions caused by HPV

Women with precancerous lesions, cervical cancer or vulvar cancer, have an increased risk for anal cancer.

The causal factor (HPV) is present in the anal-genital area, and the body has a relative sensitivity.

Smoking

Smoking is considered a contributing factor and we recommend quitting it. Smokers have more recurrences of precancerous lesions after treatment.

Cervical cancer

244. What is the frequency of cervical cancer?

The incidence of cervical cancer varies from country to country.

In countries with organized prevention systems, where women are screened at regular intervals, precancerous lesions are detected and treated. In these countries, the incidence of cervical cancer is relatively low.

Statistical data from the USA show that approximately 11,000-12,000 new cervical cancer cases appear each year, resulting in 4,000-4,500 deaths from the disease. In European countries, around 35,000 new cases are reported each year, resulting in 17,000 women losing their life from the disease.

In developing countries, the incidence of cervical cancer is very high. It is estimated that, across the globe, there are 500,000 new cases every year and 240,000 deaths.

245. Which types of HPV cause cervical cancer more frequently?

90% of cervical cancer cases are caused by HPV 16, 18, 31 33, 45, 52 and 58. HPV 16 and 18 cause 70% of cancers.

246. At what age does it usually affect women?

Cervical cancer usually appears in relatively young women. It is the second most frequent cancer in women younger than 44.

CANCERS CAUSED BY GENITAL TYPES OF HPV

247. Which women are at a higher risk for cervical cancer?
The following parameters increase the risk for cervical cancer:
- Multiple sexual partners, or a partner with a large number of sexual partners in their history (it increases the risk of becoming infected with oncogenic types of HPV).
- Starting sexual activity at a young age (<18 years).
- Personal history of precancerous lesions in the lower reproductive system.
- Smoking.
- History of other sexually transmitted infections (e.g. chlamydia).
- Poor function of the immune system.
- A family history of cervical cancer.

248. Does cervical cancer develop overnight?
No. It usually takes several years. Precancerous lesions (HSIL/CIN2, 3) appear first and cancer develops later (see figures a-h, pages 160-161).

249. What are the symptoms of cervical cancer?
Its symptoms may be:
- Vaginal bleeding after intercourse
- Increase of blood quantity during menstruation
- Bloody vaginal discharge
- Odorous vaginal discharge, sometimes with blood traces

In cases of advanced cervical cancer, there may be: pelvic pain, difficulty urinating, swollen feet, swollen lymph nodes, etc.

250. How is cervical cancer diagnosis made?

Diagnosis always requires a biopsy.

Once cervical cancer is diagnosed on biopsy, the physician will assess the size of the tumor and the extent of the disease. In addition to the gynecological pelvic examination (Figure 15, p. 203), we may also perform a rectal digital palpation, CT scan, MRI, cystoscopy, colonoscopy and other tests to find if cancer has spread to other organs.

251. What is staging?

Staging is applied to all cancers. It is the process of grading the severity of the disease based on its dispersion in the body. The lower the stage, the less advanced the disease.

Stage 0 is the stage of non-invasive carcinoma, also referred to as carcinoma in situ. At this stage, cancer cells are found only inside the epithelium of the cervix. There is no risk of metastasis.

Invasive cervical cancer (as most cancers) is classified in 4 stages (I, II, III, and IV).

Stages of invasive cervical cancer:
- The cancer has spread from the cervix lining (mucosa) into the deeper tissue but is still only found in the cervix. It has not spread to lymph nodes or other parts of the body.
- The cancer has grown beyond the uterus but not to the pelvic wall or to the lower third of the vagina.
- The tumor extends to the pelvic wall, and/or involves the lower third of the vagina, but has not spread to the lymph nodes or other parts of the body.
- The cancer has spread to the bladder or rectum and may or may not have spread to the lymph nodes or other parts of the body.

During the process of grading the severity of the disease your doctor must find:
- Where the tumor is located in the body
- The size of the tumor
- Whether cancer has spread to a different part of the body
- Whether cancer has spread to nearby lymph nodes
- The cell type (such as adenocarcinoma or squamous cell carcinoma)
- Tumor grade, which refers to how abnormal the cancer cells look and how likely the tumor is to grow and spread.

FIGURE 15: Palpation during a pelvic exam

Palpation: The doctor inserts two fingers (usually the index and middle finger) of one hand into the vagina, and with the other hand applies pressure on the abdomen from the outside, trying to palpate the internal genital organs.

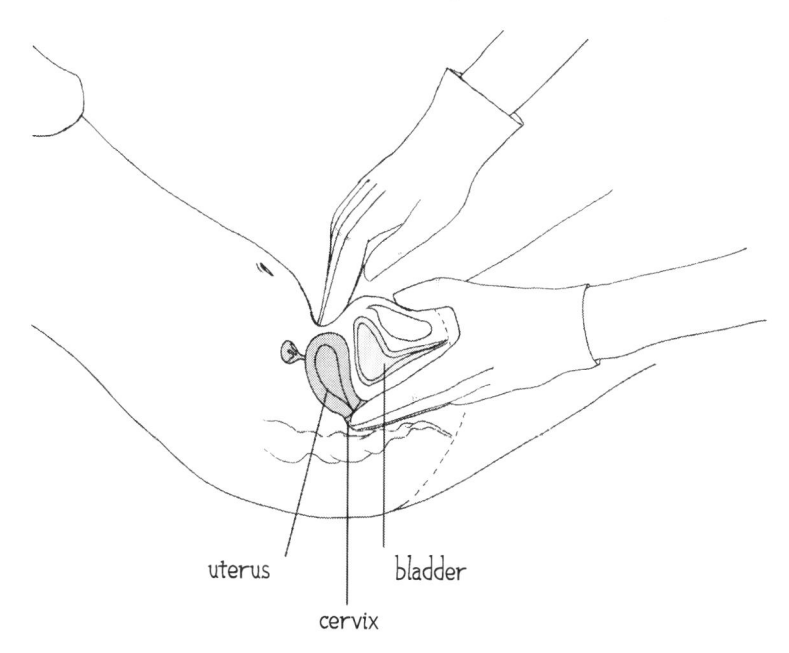

252. What is metastasis?

In cases with invasive cancer, cancer cells have broken through the basal membrane of the epithelium and have entered deep into the cervical tissue that is full of blood and lymphatic vessels. Blood and lymphatic vessels are eroded by cancer, and cancer cells start, from this point onward, to travel far from their original focus (the cervix) and take residence in other organs of the body, where they create secondary tumors (metastases).

Cancer spreads in 3 ways.
- Local spreading (cancer spreads to neighboring tissues and organs).
- Spreading through lymphatic vessels, initially to neighboring lymph nodes, and then to other parts of the body and
- Spreading through blood vessels to distant organs (e.g. lungs, bones, liver, etc.).

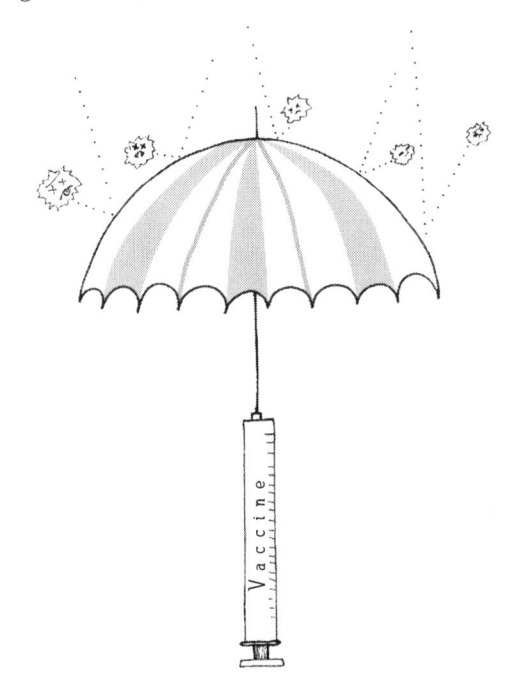

253. What are the treatments for cervical cancer?

Treatment depends on the stage of the disease.
There are three treatment methods:
- Radical hysterectomy
- Radiation therapy and
- Chemotherapy

A combination of treatment methods is frequently chosen, in order to achieve the best result.

254. What is the prognosis for invasive cervical cancer?

As seen in Table 6, the rates for five-year survival drop for the higher stages of cervical cancer.

255. How successful is the prevention of cervical cancer?

Chapters 1-6 describe in detail the preventive measures, which, if correctly implemented (combination of vaccination at a young age and secondary prevention later with Pap tests and/or HPV tests), can prevent cervical cancer at rates close to 100%.

TABLE 6

The stages of cervical cancer and 5-year survival rates

Stage	Five-year survival
I	80%-90%
II	65%-70%
III	40%
IV	20%

HPV-related vaginal cancer

256. How common is vaginal cancer?
Vaginal cancer is rarer compared to cervical and vulvar cancer.

257. Is HPV the cause of vaginal cancer?
A percentage of vaginal cancers is caused by oncogenic types of HPV (60%). These cancers that are caused by HPV are usually preceded by premalignant lesions (HSIL/VaIN 2, 3).

258. Which women are at a higher risk for vaginal cancer?
At risk for precancerous lesions and HPV-related vaginal cancers are:
- Women with a history of cervical precancerous lesions or cervical cancer.
- Women who have had their uterus removed due to cervical precancerous lesions or cervical cancer.
- Women with precancerous lesions or HPV-related cancer in the vulva and anus.

The risk for carcinogenesis in the vagina from HPV increases in smokers and women under immunosuppression.

259. What about vaginal cancer prevention measures?
Prevention includes vaccination and check-ups.

There are no special prevention programs for vaginal cancer (like there are for cervical cancer) because it is a rare cancer in the general population.

However, it is recommended that women with a history of precancerous lesions or cancer in the lower genital tract are also preventively examined in the vagina, even if their uterus has been removed.

260. What is the treatment of vaginal cancer?
Treatment consists of the surgical removal of the vagina (colpectomy), partial or total, in combination with radiation therapy.

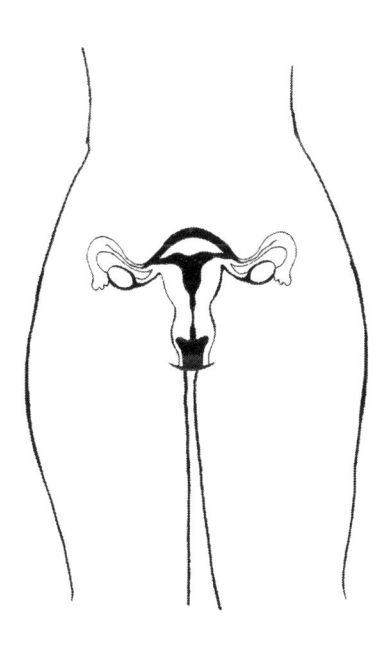

HPV-related vulvar cancer

261. How common is vulvar cancer?
Vulvar cancer is not particularly common.

According to the American Cancer Society, 4850 vulvar cancer cases were reported in 2014 in the USA.

262. What percentage of vulvar cancers is attributed to oncogenic types of HPV?
It is believed that 40% of vulvar cancers are related to HPV. The statistical data from Europe and the USA show that there is a rise in HPV-related vulvar cancers, attributed to the epidemic of HPV infections.

263. What factors increase the chance of HPV-related vulvar cancer?
- A history of precancerous lesions (VIN) or other intraepithelial neoplasia or HPV-related cancer in the lower genital tract or the anal area
- A history of genital warts
- Age. The risk increases in a woman's fourth decade and onwards.

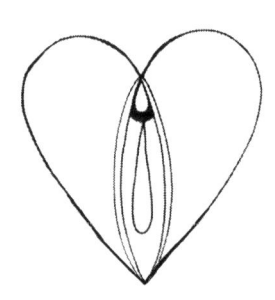

- Smoking. In women with a history of infection from oncogenic types of HPV, smoking increases the risk for carcinogenesis in the vulva.

264. What are the symptoms, what does it look like?

In the beginning, vulvar cancer caused by HPV causes no symptoms. The lesion later looks like:
- an ulcer (wound) or
- protrusion or lump on the skin or
- like a harder area with "tension".

The color of the lesion may be lighter or darker than the skin of the vulva or look pink or red.

265. What does diagnosis entail?

Diagnosis is made with a clinical examination and a biopsy.

266. What happens after the initial biopsy?

Staging follows the histological diagnosis. Staging requires, apart from the pelvic examination, a series of other examinations, like colposcopy, cystoscopy, anoscopy, chest X-ray, CT scan, etc.

267. How is vulvar cancer treated?

There are different treatments depending on the cancer stage.

The three main treatment methods are:
- surgical treatment
- radiation therapy
- chemotherapy

Vulvar cancer in the early stages is treated surgically, while, in more advanced stages, a combination of the above methods is used.

268. Why should VIN lesions be found and treated?

HPV-related squamous cell carcinoma of the vulva usually forms slowly over many years. Precancerous changes (VIN) often occur first and can last for several years.

Women with VIN lesions have an increased risk of developing invasive vulvar cancer.

The risk of progression to cancer seems to be highest with VIN 3 lesions. This risk can be altered with treatment. In one study, 88% of untreated VIN3 progressed to cancer, whereas only 4% of the women who were treated developed vulvar cancer.

269. Can HPV-related vulvar cancers be prevented?

The majority of these cancers are prevented if the following measures are taken:
- Preventive measures to reduce the risk of HPV infection (vaccination, use of a condom, limitation of sexual partners).
- Check-ups, especially in women with an HPV infection history, in order to detect in time any precancerous lesions (VIN).
- Quitting smoking.

Anal cancer

270. What is the cause of anal cancer?

The majority of anal cancers are caused by oncogenic types of HPV.

271. How common is anal cancer?

Cancers of the anal canal are currently 4% of all cancers of the large intestine. It is not, therefore, a common cancer. However, there has been an increase in the incidence of HPV-related anal cancer.

According to the American Cancer Society, there were 7210 new anal cancer cases in 2014. Of these, 4550 cases were in women and 2660 in men.

It is estimated that the risk for anal cancer in one's lifetime is 1:500 in the general population. As the above statistical data show, the risk is higher in women compared to men. It appears, however, that certain individuals are at a greater risk of anal cancer.

272. At what age does anal cancer usually appear?

Anal cancer is rare in people younger than 35 years of age. It mainly affects adults, above the age of 50. The average age at diagnosis is 60 years.

273. What are the signs and symptoms of anal cancer?

There are usually no symptoms in early stages. Later on, there may be:
- Anal bleeding.
- Bloody discharge after anal intercourse.

- Impression or palpation of a mass in the anal canal area.
- Itching and mucous or purulent anal discharge.
- Changes in bowel movements.
- Palpation of lymph nodes.

Figure 16: Carcinogenesis from HPV in the anus
The metaplastic epithelium of the anus at the sphincter level is infected by oncogenic types of HPV. A persistent infection may lead to precancerous lesions and cancer.

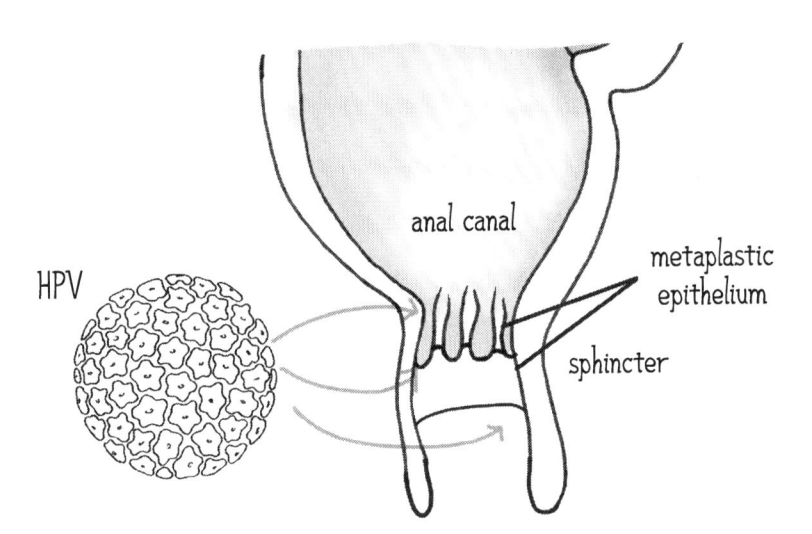

274. What is the connection between anal warts and anal cancer?
Anal warts are usually caused by HPV 6 and 11. These types of HPV are low-risk and do not cause anal cancer.

It has been observed, however, that people with a history of anal warts have a higher possibility of anal cancer. It is believed that, apart from low-risk types of HPV, they were also infected by high-risk types of HPV, and this is why they are at an increased risk (Figure 16).

275. What tests are recommended for the prevention of anal cancer?
- Clinical examination by the doctor (digital examination).
- Pap test or HPV test from the anal canal.
- High-Resolution anoscopy and biopsies.

276. Can anal cancer be prevented?
It appears that anal cancer can be prevented, and prevention programs are already under way. Vaccination before becoming sexually active can prevent 95% of HPV-related anal cancers.

Even though the physical history of carcinogenesis from HPV in the anus has not been fully clarified, it is believed that precancerous lesions usually appear first (HSIL/AIN2,3), and these must be identified and treated.

The groups referred for preventive annual check-ups are:
- HIV-positive patients (AIDS)
- Homosexual men
- Individuals with a history of anal warts
- Women with a history of HSIL in the cervix, vagina or vulva and
- Individuals under chronic pharmaceutical immunosuppression

Head and neck cancers attributed to HPV

277. What are the factors for carcinogenesis in the head and neck?

Cancers that are known collectively as head and neck cancers usually begin in the squamous cells that line the moist, mucosal surfaces inside the head and neck (for example, inside the mouth, the nose, and the throat).

The factors that are causally linked to the above cancers include smoking and excessive consumption of alcohol. In the past decade, however, oncogenic types of HPV were also linked to head and neck cancers (mostly to orophagyngeal cancers – cancers of the tonsils, base of tongue etc.).

Head and neck cancers caused by oncogenic types of HPV are constantly increasing in the USA. It is believed that a significant percentage (25-35%) of oropharyngeal cancers in the USA are currently caused by HPV (mostly by HPV16).

278. Where do HPV-related cancers usually appear?

The most common areas are around the base of the tongue and the tonsils.

279. How is HPV transmitted to the oropharynx?

It is believed that transmission takes place through oral sex. The possibility of transmission by kissing (mouth to mouth) is disputed or considered low.

Statistics show that the possibility of infections and carcinogenesis by oncogenic types of HPV increases depending on the number of sexual partners (and engaging in oral sex).

280. How common are oropharyngeal HPV infections?

Studies in the USA have shown that:
- Around 7% of the population has HPV in the oral cavity.
- However, only 1% has HPV16, which is the type more frequently implicated in oropharyngeal cancer.
- Sexually active individuals aged 14-44 reported an oral sex experience at a percentage of 80%.

281. Does HPV cause carcinogenesis in the oropharynx immediately after the infection?

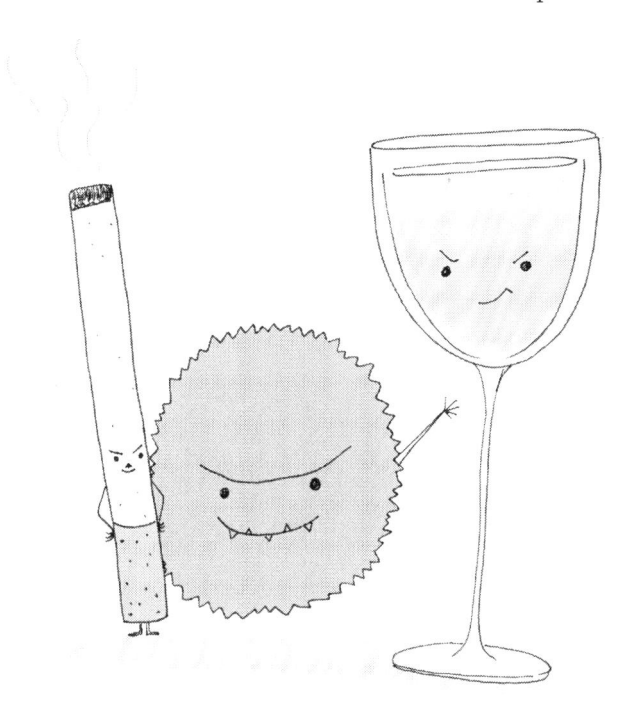

No, it appears that many years have to pass before developing into cancer. From the data we have up to now, in some people it took more than 15 years. Smoking and tobacco chewing appear to be contributing factors in carcinogenesis.

282. At what ages does oropharyngeal cancer appear?
Oropharyngeal cancer is rare prior to the age of 55. Today, the average age at diagnosis of such cancers is 62 years. However, due to the epidemic outbreak of HPV diseases and changes in sexual habits (more frequent oral sex), it is believed that cancer may appear in younger ages in the future. Oropharyngeal cancer is more common in men than women (3:1 ratio).

283. Should a couple's sex life change if an oropharyngeal HPV lesion is discovered?
Nothing needs to change in the sexual behavior of a couple in a long-term relationship. We know that, in long-term relationships, both partners have usually been infected.

284. What prevention measures can be taken for oropharyngeal cancer?
- Preventive HPV vaccination (best before becoming sexually active).
- Restriction of the number, and careful selection of sexual partners.
- Avoiding smoking and excessive consumption of alcohol.
- Care for maintaining a healthy immune system.

285. Is there any test that finds lesions?
There is no test to date that is used to prevent oropharyngeal cancer (similar to the Pap and HPV tests).

286. How can you find out if you should be concerned about any symptom you are experiencing?

If you have symptoms or observe something out of the ordinary you can see an ENT (Ear – Nose – Throat) doctor. Also, your dentist can guide you and refer you to an oral medicine specialist if you feel that you have a problem inside the oral cavity.

You must seek the opinion of a specialist if you see anything suspicious, such as:
- Wound or ulcer that does not heal within 2-3 weeks
- Swelling in the area
- Difficulty swallowing
- Pain during chewing
- Irritated throat, coarseness, coughing

CHAPTER 11

Men and HPV (everything your partner would like to know)

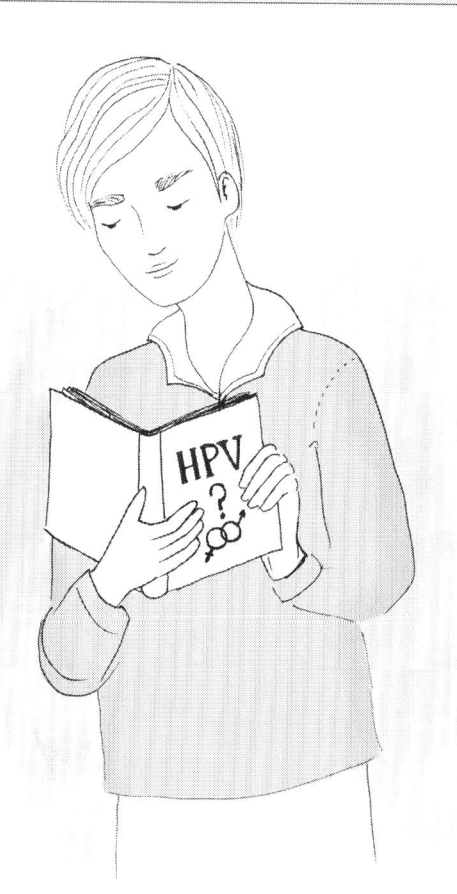

Transmission of the infection and effects on men

287. How common are infections from genital types of HPV in men?

According to the current epidemiological data and modern habits in the western world (frequent change of sexual partners in young ages), it is estimated that nearly all sexually active men are infected by certain genital types of HPV over their lifetime. In most cases, temporary local lesions are created, which go unnoticed and subside on their own within a few months. In some cases, however, there are visible genital warts. In very few cases, precancerous lesions may appear much later.

288. How are genital types of HPV transmitted in men?

Genital types of HPV are transmitted through sexual intercourse. In the first chapter (page 69) we described in detail the transmission of genital types of HPV. A man may reduce the risk of infection by consistently using condoms throughout the entire duration of intercourse.

289. What do genital types of HPV cause in men?

After the infection, genital types of HPV may cause lesions, if the immune system allows it.

Most of these lesions are invisible and cause no symptoms. They are, therefore, called subclinical. In some cases, visible lesions appear, referred to as genital warts.

A long time after the infection and the first lesions by oncogenic types of HPV, there is a small chance of precancerous lesions appearing.

Infections are common but cancer is rare. There is a correlation with the type of the virus. Precancerous lesions and cancers are only caused by oncogenic types of HPV.

We describe below, in order of frequency, the lesions caused by genital types of HPV in men:
- Subclinical lesions
- Genital warts
- Precancerous lesions and cancer.

Subclinical (invisible) lesions

As we described in the first chapter (p. 57), most lesions are subclinical (cannot be found during a clinical examination, are invisible to the naked eye, and cause no symptoms). Throughout the duration of a subclinical infection, the man transmits the infection to his partner without being aware of it.

All genital types of HPV can cause subclinical lesions.

Subclinical lesions have a good prognosis. They subside on their own within a few months. No treatment is recommended for subclinical lesions but it is possible that they will recur.

Genital warts

Genital warts, referred to as condylomata accuminata in the medical texts, are benign infectious lesions and nearly 90% of them are caused by HPV 6 and 11. Other genital types of HPV are responsible for the remaining 10%.

About 1-3% of the male population will get genital warts by the age of 50. It is obvious that there is a higher possibility of genital warts in men:
- who have sex with a person suffering from genital warts
- who have sex with a person with a history of genital warts
- who have a history with a large number of sexual partners.

The possibility of transmission of the virus and appearance of genital warts is very high in those cases where at the time of sexual contact, the partner has genital warts (60-70% risk of transmission).

As regards the detection of genital warts in men, they usually appear on the penis. Less frequently, they appear on the pubis, scrotum, groin, and the perianal area (more frequently in homosexuals receiving anal intercourse). Perianal warts have been found in men with warts in the genital organs who have had no anal intercourse, obviously due to self-infection (see autoinoculation, p. 70).

Genital warts cause no serious symptoms. Several patients report itching.

DON'T FORGET

Genital warts, as a rule, are benign. The recommendation, however, is to treat them because they are highly infectious and, in many cases, cause functional, aesthetic, and psychological problems.

Precancerous lesions and cancer

In very few cases, and a long time after the initial infection with oncogenic types of HPV, precancerous lesions may appear. If precancerous lesions are not treated, they may develop into cancer.

In men, precancerous lesions and cancers caused by HPV have been described on the penis and anal area. Also, it is estimated that 25%-35% of head and neck cancers (oral cavity and throat) are attributed to genital types of HPV.

Precancerous lesions on the penis are internationally referred to with the initials PeIN (Penile Intraepithelial Neoplasia). The corresponding term used for precancerous anal lesions is AIN (Anal Intraepithelial Neoplasia). There are grades AIN 1, 2, 3 corresponding to the CIN, VIN, and VaIN lesions described in chapters 8 and 9. It is believed that AIN 2/3 lesions (also referred to as HSIL) must be treated because there is a significant chance that they will develop into cancer.

Penile cancer: Penile cancer is exceptionally rare. However, a large percentage (40%-50%) of penile cancers is causally related to infection by oncogenic types of HPV. Around 600 penile cancers are reported every year in the USA (0.2% of cancers in men). Due to the rarity of the disease, no routine check-up is recommended. However, if any precancerous lesions are found on the penis, they must, of course, be treated.

As regards anal cancer in men: around 2,000 anal cancer cases are reported every year in the United States. Approximately 95% of anal cancers are attributed to HPV.

We know that, in male homosexuals, high-risk types of HPV cause precancerous lesions and cancer of the anal canal more frequently. AIDS patients are at a higher risk for carcinogenesis due to immunosuppression. There are efforts to establish routine check-ups for male homosexuals, with tests similar to those for the prevention of cervical cancer in women (Pap test and HPV test).

Finally, in regard to head and neck cancers: High-risk types of HPV are responsible for carcinogenesis in the mouth, pharynx, and larynx areas (described as head and neck cancers). The DNA of oncogenic types of HPV is found in 25%-35% of the cancers in these areas (usually HPV 16).

Head and neck cancers are not very common, and most of them appear in men after the age of 50. Smoking and alcohol abuse have always been considered causal factors. However, it is important to acknowledge that even some of these cancers are caused by oncogenic types of HPV, because they could be prevented with HPV vaccination in boys.

290. Which factors affect the risk of a man getting infected by HPV?

The risk increases with the number of sexual partners and the sexual history of each partner.

The risk decreases with the use of condoms.

Preventive vaccination, before becoming sexually active, provides a high rate of protection. It provides nearly 100% protection against the vaccine's HPV types.

It is also worth noting that circumcised men have a smaller chance of chronic HPV penile infections. This does not mean that circumcision fully protects from the risk of infection. How is this explained? In circumcised men, the glans of the penis is not covered by the foreskin, the area is dry, and the epithelium is covered by keratin. In these conditions, it is not easy for HPV to cause chronic infections, because, as we described in the first chapter, HPV prefers moist areas with metaplastic epithelium.

Diagnosis and treatment

291. What are the symptoms of a man recently infected with HPV?

As we already mentioned, the majority of HPV infected men have only subclinical (not visible) lesions which are not usually accompanied by any symptoms, and therefore go unnoticed. Only genital warts are noticed, because they are visible.

292. How are genital warts diagnosed?

Genital warts are usually visible by the patient, who seeks a medical opinion. Diagnosis is based on clinical examination, that is assisted by the use of a magnifying glass. In very few cases is a biopsy required to confirm the diagnosis.

293. How are subclinical infections and precancerous lesions diagnosed?

Subclinical lesions are by definition not visible to the naked eye. A section of the tissue (biopsy) must be examined under the microscope and the epithelium must be studied, in order to diagnose them. This procedure is not generally recommended for detecting simple infections, since they usually subside on their own.

Biopsies are taken when precancerous lesions are suspected on the penis and anus. The location of the biopsy is decided by the doctor. An acetic acid solution is frequently used, the same one used during colposcopy for women.

The anal canal is checked with the use of a colposcope and an acetic acid solution (the same technique with the colposcopy - see p. 118). The examination is internationally referred to as a "high-resolution anoscopy."

A high-resolution anoscopy is recommended in cases of anal warts, especially in immunosuppressed patients.

294. Can a man be tested to find out if he has been infected with HPV in the past?

As we mentioned before many times, most infections from HPV go unnoticed and subside spontaneously. As long as an HPV infection is active on the epithelium, the doctor may take a biopsy and confirm it under a microscope. After the lesions subside, there is nothing visible, not even under a microscope. There is also no test for detecting HPV antibodies in the blood, like there is for other viruses (herpes, etc.). There is no diagnostic test, therefore, to find out whether someone was once infected, unless he reports genital warts in his history.

An active HPV infection on the cervix can be detected with a Pap test and an HPV test. A similar process can be used by collecting material from the anal canal. This does not apply, however, to the penis area, because it is impossible to collect appropriate material and the results of the test are considered unreliable.

295. What treatment should men get?

No treatment is recommended for subclinical infections.

Only genital warts, precancerous lesions, and, of course, the rare cases of cancer are treated.

Genital wart treatment

Patients are initially advised to quit smoking, because smoking affects the immune system and decreases the success rates of the treatment, while it increases recurrence rates.

The treatment methods are those described in chapter 7.

Precancerous lesion treatment

Precancerous lesions in male genital organs and the anus are treated the same way as similar lesions in women (question 236, p. 193). The lesions are destroyed or removed if a detailed examination of the tissue under a microscope is required to exclude the possibility of invasive cancer.

Prevention

296. Is there any preventive test for penile cancer in men?

Penile cancer is more frequent in older men.

It is a very rare cancer, and there are, therefore, no recommendations for screening of the male population with any routine test. However, in any case where a man notices any change on his penis or displays any symptoms, he should consult his doctor. Most precancerous lesions on the penis are visible and found by the patients themselves. The color of the lesions varies (white, gray, brown, red). The lesions may be small and dispersed or there may be a solitary large lesion (diameter > 1cm). Solitary lesions are more serious when it comes to their prognosis. Lesions are more frequently found on the glans of the penis.

297. Is there any preventive test for anal cancer in men?

The only category of men who should be checked is men with a history of receptive anal intercourse, especially immunosuppressed men. The observation that anal cancer is 17 times more frequent in male homosexuals (especially when there is a concurrent HIV infection the risk is much higher), led American researchers to study precancerous anal lesions and anal cancer in more detail.

There is metaplastic epithelium on the anal canal, similar to the cervix, located between the cylindrical epithelium of the rectum and the squamous epithelium covering the entrance of the anal canal. Precancerous lesions and cancers caused by oncogenic types of HPV usually appear in the area with the metaplastic epithelium. It was found that a preventive Pap test or an HPV test from the anal canal will frequently detect precancerous lesions. It has not been clarified however, if finding and treating precancerous lesions contributes toward decreasing anal cancers, therefore no official recommendation by scientific societies has been made yet in order to institute this method.

298. Can an HPV infection be prevented in men?

There are around 40 different genital types of HPV that infect genital organs and the anal area. Infections caused in the population by the transmission of these types of HPV during sex are very frequent. The transmissibility of the infection from one person to another is very high.

The only way to completely avoid infection by genital types of HPV is to never have any sexual contacts. This is not, however, a reasonable choice.

The use of a condom during intercourse does not offer 100% coverage, but it does significantly reduce the risk of infection and is therefore recommended.

Certain protection from specific types of HPV is offered only by the available vaccines. It is not possible, however, to produce a vaccine protecting against all genital HPV types. Therefore, the available vaccines have been manufactured to protect from the types of HPV that cause the most frequent and serious problems.

HPV vaccines are preventive. It is recommended that boys and girls aged 11-12 years old are vaccinated as a prevention. Preventive vaccination may be carried out at older ages (there have been studies that prove the efficacy of the vaccines and their safety in ages up to 26 years old). Ages 11-12 are considered ideal for vaccination, before any sexual activity has started and, therefore, before any potential infection by certain types of HPV.

Answers to the questions of the male partner

299. Should the partner of a woman who was found with HPV infection be checked?

Both women and men may become infected by HPV during sexual intercourse, and then infect their next partners. This is the rule in the majority of cases, because there are usually no visible lesions, only subclinical ones, and individuals infected with HPV are not aware of it.

Old infections become latent and may be activated again. When an infection is latent, neither men nor women are infectious. However, if at some point the immune system is suppressed, the virus is activated again and lesions reappear, presenting a renewed risk of transmission to the partner.

If genital warts are found in a woman, the recommendation is that her partner is also checked as a precaution. Men who see any lesions on their penis should also be examined. No routine examination is recommended for men simply because their partner was found with a subclinical HPV infection.

300. My partner was diagnosed with an HPV infection. What are the risks for my health?

Usually, both partners are infected, especially in long-term relationships.

If your partner was diagnosed with genital warts and you don't have any, you should avoid any sexual contact until she gets treated and warts have disappeared. Optionally, you may be examined by a doctor in the event you have any unnoticed lesions.

If subclinical HPV lesions were diagnosed in your partner (by a Pap test, HPV test or a colposcopy) and you have no symptoms, it is not recommended that you do anything. You can, of course, get examined if you so wish, but there are no immediate risks to your health.

CHAPTER 12

You and HPV – You don't need to worry if…

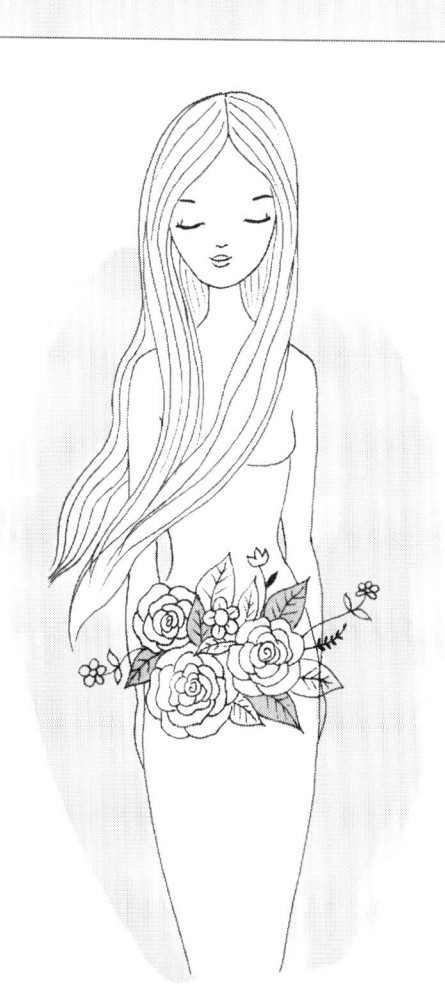

The effects from genital types of HPV on you and your children

301. What are the general problems in the population?

HPV infections are the most common sexually transmitted infections, with significant effects on the population. As we described in previous chapters, the diseases caused by HPV are numerous and affect both men and women.

Except for the (benign and malignant) diseases caused, there are several psychological effects from these infections, as well as an economic cost for society (around 8 billion dollars annually in the USA).

302. What are the psychological consequences when a woman finds out she has been infected?

As a rule, women begin to worry when they find out that they have been infected with HPV. The infection is perceived by the woman as a triple risk: a risk for her life, a risk for her fertility, and a risk for her relationship with her partner.

Most women believe that they did something wrong and got sexually infected by a virus that can cause cancer. They get stressed and have strong negative feelings, such as:

- Fear and concern for their life and fertility.
- Disappointment, and sometimes despair, because there is no permanent cure to rid them completely of the virus.
- Remorse, because a sexually transmitted disease carries a stigma for many people.

303. What questions do couples have after a positive diagnosis of an HPV infection? What should the doctor do?

Diagnosis of an infection in either partner usually gives rise to questions such as:
- Who infected whom?
- Is my partner having an affair?
- Does my partner continue to transmit the virus?
- Is it possible that I had the virus beforehand?
- How can we find out what really happened?

The doctor's role is to try to prevent and relieve as much as possible the emotional reactions, the psychological and social consequences, and to provide answers to the couple's questions (the above questions have been answered in the book's previous pages).

Don't feel bad – Overcome your fears
Be informed – Knowledge is power!

304. Is there any reason to feel bad because your doctor told you that have been infected with HPV?

There is no reason to have any negative feelings. You are not alone in having been infected with HPV.

HPV infection is very common. It is estimated that more than 80% of the population may become infected with one or more types of HPV over their lifetime. You are not alone in this. You just didn't know it.

HPV lives parasitically in the epithelium of the genital organs. Most people infected with HPV don't know it because they have no visible lesions or symptoms. You can't know if the DNA of some of the 40 genital types of HPV is inside the cells of the genital organs of your partner. He is not aware of it either. There is nothing you or your partner did wrong.

Do not worry. The vast majority of lesions that appear usually subside on their own. Even if there are some problems, modern medicine can successfully address them. You must not, therefore, feel bad; you are not alone. It is simply best to get regular check-ups, according to the recommendations of your doctor.

The real issue is not your past behavior. You can't change that. What you can control is your health and practices in the present and future. You have the power to monitor your health, keep the HPV under control, and prevent HPV-related diseases.

305. What basic knowledge must every woman have?

There are around 40 different genital types of HPV that infect women and men. These are mainly transmitted through sexual contact. They are distinguished between low and high-risk because they may cause benign or malignant diseases.

- Genital warts usually caused by low-risk types of HPV may be annoying, but do not develop into cancer.
- Cancer is caused by high-risk types of HPV. This is considered a rare possibility with a common infection, and most cases of cancer are prevented.
- There is no cure for HPV. Like the flu, it's a virus and can't be treated with antibiotics. Because this is the case, prevention is always the best defense.

- There are two methods of prevention. The first is to get vaccinated preventively and not allow the virus to infect you. The second is to detect any precancerous lesions and treat them before they develop into cancer. Getting vaccinated and scheduling regular check-ups will go a long way toward minimizing any woman's risk.
- It is impossible to develop a vaccine that will cover all genital types of HPV. The vaccines that have been developed, however, will protect you against the types of HPV that cause the most frequent problems. These vaccines protect you from the specific types of HPV if you get vaccinated before becoming infected.
- The most common cancer caused by HPV in women is cervical cancer. Thankfully, it can be prevented because precancerous lesions usually precede cancer, which appears later. It is, therefore, necessary to get regular check-ups in order to detect any precancerous lesions and treat them.
- The check-up currently used for cervical cancer is very successful and reliable. In addition to the Pap test, there is also the HPV test, which detects infection from oncogenic types of HPV. The reliability of the latter is higher than 90%. In cases where the check-up comes up with positive findings, it is followed by a colposcopy and biopsies.
- Vaccination of girls (before the start of any sexual activity) in combination with check-ups for cervical cancer (regular check-ups in women) are considered to protect women from specific types of cancer at rates very close to 100%!

- As regards the other cancers caused by HPV, your doctor will inform you how you can prevent them. It is believed that the vaccination of children at an age around 11 or 12 will protect them from the majority of these cancers (90%).

306. What should you do to protect your children?

All the scientific data available has shown that the vaccination of children before the start of any sexual activity has certain and significant advantages. It is recommended that both girls and boys are vaccinated at ages 11-12.

307. You were diagnosed with an HPV infection. Is there any risk of infecting your children?

Genital types of HPV are transmitted as a rule through sexual intercourse. One must come in contact with skin or mucous membranes with HPV lesions to become infected with the virus. There is, therefore, no reason for concern for your children.

308. How should you manage an HPV infection together with your partner?

Do not let it affect your peace or happiness. Ask an expert for information. Make sure you are correctly informed on the subject. It is usually uncertain which partner infected the other (unless one of the two had never had a relationship in the past).

It is not possible to know exactly when and by whom one became infected. Both women and men may become infected by HPV during sexual intercourse, and then infect their next partners. This is the rule in the majority of cases, because no visible lesions are usually present, only subclinical ones, and individuals infected with HPV are not aware of it.

Unfair though it seems, there isn't an approved HPV test for males. Only people with a history of genital warts know that they were once infected. However, even these individuals don't know if they have been infected with oncogenic types of HPV. Also, they may believe they were cured and no longer carry the virus.

Old infections become latent, and may be activated again. When an infection is latent, neither men nor women are infectious. If at some point in the future the immune system is suppressed, the virus is reactivated and lesions reappear, presenting a risk of transmission to the partner.

In long-term relationships, usually both partners have been infected. Your partner may not have any lesions at this time (if he is examined), but this does not mean that there is no HPV DNA in his cells. His immune system is simply working properly and has suppressed the infection. Several studies indicate that "shared HPV" does not "ping pong" back and forth. There is evidence, though, that when lesions are found in one partner, using condoms may speed the clearance of any HPV-related disease. The decreased viral load may allow the individual's own immune system a better chance of eliminating the virus.

Boost your defense mechanisms with a healthy lifestyle

309. What is the role of your defense mechanisms in carcinogenesis?

It has been proven that a persistent HPV infection caused by high-risk viral types over a long period of time increases the chances for cancer in the future.

What factors contribute to the persistence of an HPV infection and carcinogenesis later? The deficient functioning of our immune system and the tumor-suppressing mechanisms we have (if they don't work properly).

The poor functioning of our immune system, whatever its cause, is a very important parameter. We know that AIDS patients are at a higher risk due to the deficient functioning of their immune system. Also, as we know, patients taking immunosuppressant medication for any reason (such as organ transplant patients, chronic users of cortisone and other immunosuppressive drugs due to rheumatism or other chronic diseases) face a higher risk.

High-risk HPVs drive abnormal cell proliferation, as a consequence of genetic alterations, and induce mutations.

Once HPV enters an epithelial cell, the virus begins to make the proteins it encodes. Two of the proteins made by high-risk HPVs (E6 and E7) interfere with cell functions that normally prevent excessive growth, helping the mutated cells to grow in an uncontrolled manner and to avoid cell death.

Many times the HPV infected cells are recognized by the immune system and eliminated. Sometimes, however, these infected cells are not destroyed, resulting in a persistent infection. As the persistently infected cells continue to multiply, they may develop mutations in cellular genes that promote even more abnormal cell growth, leading to the formation of an area of precancerous cells and, ultimately, a cancerous tumor.

There are also genetic factors (hereditary) that determine how well these mechanisms work in each one of us. We have not yet managed to uncover many details on this subject. These two parameters must, of course, be taken into consideration, i.e. age (the older an individual is, the greater the risk for carcinogenesis) and the family history of cancer.

310. What can you do to improve your immune system?

In order to improve your immune system, you should:
- avoid stress
- get adequate sleep
- quit smoking
- treat other infections and
- eat a healthy diet (with green vegetables and plenty of fruit - to get vitamins A, B, E, C. Foods rich in Omega3 fats and the consumption of green tea are also recommended).

311. Why is it good not to smoke?

In addition to its other harmful effects on our health, smoking weakens our defense mechanisms against HPV.

It reduces the action of certain cells of our immune system (such as the Langerhans cells) that are responsible for the suppression of the virus, at a local level in the tissues of the lower genital tract.

It has also been proven that the cancer-causing substances of tobacco (such as benzopyrene, cotinine, phenols, etc.) are detected in the mucus of a smoker's cervix (in a concentration many times higher than the blood) and may act as contributing factors in carcinogenesis.

It appears that smoking has an especially aggravating effect on the suppression of HPV activity by the woman's body and on how it fights carcinogenesis.

As has been proven by numerous medical studies (published since 1990), smokers are at a much higher risk for recurrences of genital warts as well as precancerous lesions.

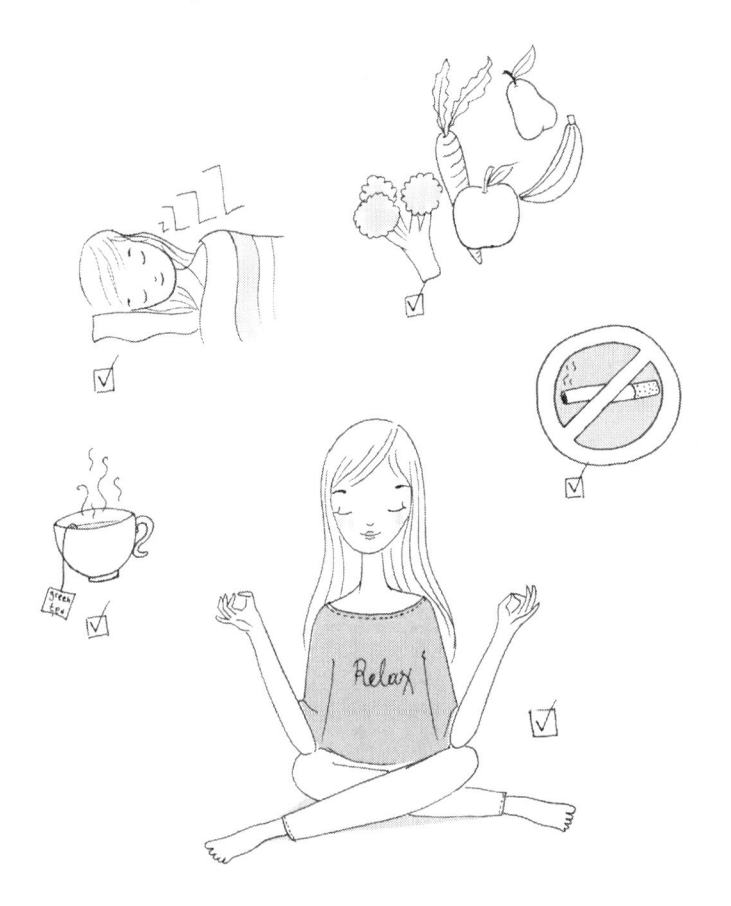

AFTERWORD

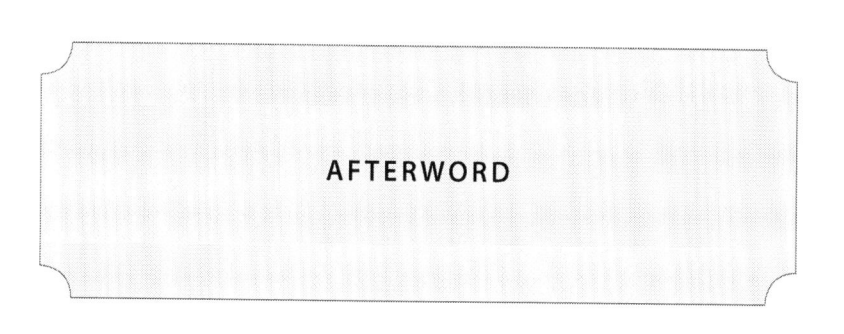

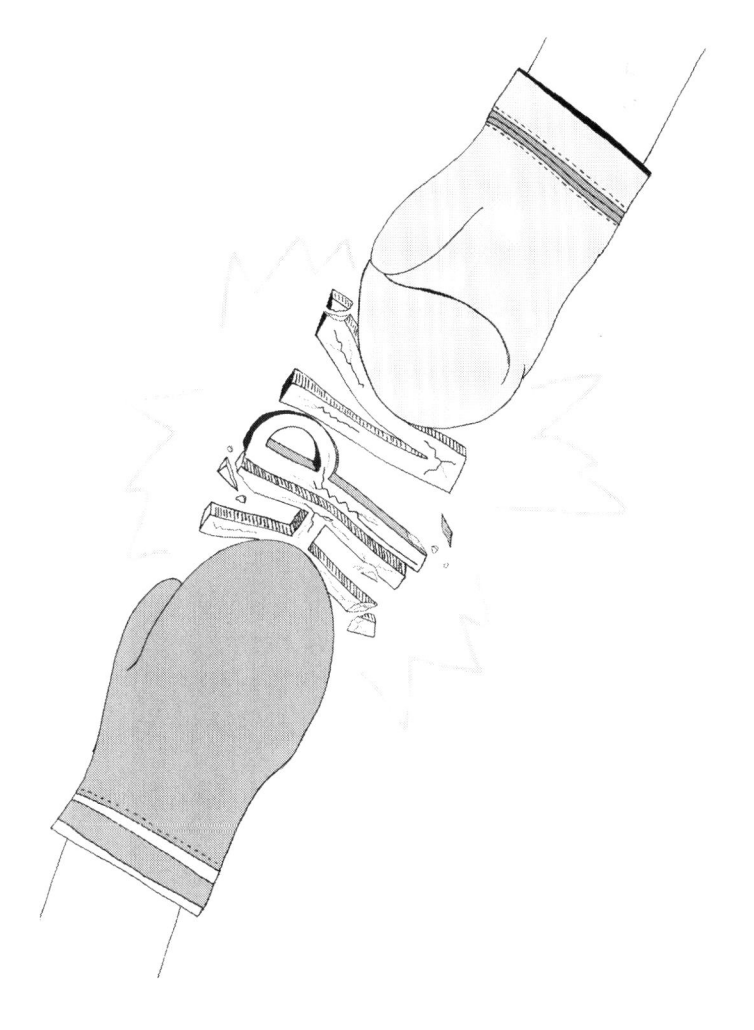

Now that you have read most of this book, I believe that your anxiety has lessened. Our fear always diminishes if we learn how to prevent or how to address a health problem.

As you found out by reading this book, there is a way to prevent most of the problems that may be caused by certain types of HPV in you or your children.

Scientific data support that the preventive administration of the Gardasil 9 vaccine to both boys and girls aged 11-12 years old will result in the reduction of HPV-related diseases by up to 90%.

Even if you did not get the vaccine yourself and have been infected with HPV, it is better that you adopt a positive view about it: the diagnosis of an HPV infection is a good opportunity to get a proper check-up and to continue getting periodical check-ups. If you do this, nothing bad can happen to you.

My personal experience from tens of thousands of cases is that women who were diagnosed with an HPV infection are lucky, because they start getting regular check-ups and eliminate the chance of cancer in the lower genital tract since, in the few cases where precancerous lesions were found, these were treated in time.

I can assure you that, in the 28 years that I have been working on this subject, among all women who initially consulted me because of an HPV infection and then continued to get check-ups every year, there was not a single one where the cancer was not diagnosed in time in the lower genital tract.

Not a single one lost her life, and only in very rare cases did we have to remove the uterus.

It is also very interesting to note that, during all these years, women who came for their annual gynecological check-ups were diagnosed with other problems, unrelated to HPV, and many lives were saved.

I am telling you this in all honesty: maybe an infection with an HPV today is a good opportunity to start getting regular check-ups and ensure your excellent health in the future. Maybe you feel uncomfortable. I know what you are thinking. That you were infected by a virus that is sexually transmitted and may cause cancer...

You are wondering what you did wrong. There is no need to feel bad, because you did nothing wrong. And you will be at no risk if you follow the instructions your doctor gives you.

BIBLIOGRAPHY

Agorastos T, Chatzistamatiou K, Katsamagkas T, et al. Primary screening for cervical cancer based on high-risk human papillomavirus (HPV) detection and HPV 16 and HPV 18 genotyping, in comparison to cytology. PLoS One. 2015; 10(3).

American Cancer Society. Cancer Facts & Figures 2014. Atlanta Am Cancer Soc. 2014. http://www.cancer.org/acs/groups/content/@research/documents/webcontent/acspc-042151.pdf.

American Cancer Society. HPV Vaccines.http://www.cancer.org/cancer-causes/othercarcinogens/infectiousagents/hpv/humanpapillomavirusandhpvvaccinesfaq/index. Accessed November 30, 2015.

American College of Pediatricians – January 2016: New concerns about the human papilloma virus vaccine. https://www.acpeds.org/the-college-speaks/position-statements/health-issues/new-concerns-about-the-human-papillomavirus-vaccine. Accessed Sept. 2nd 2016.

Arbyn M, Snijders PJF, Meijer CJLM, et al. Which high-risk HPV assays fulfil criteria for use in primary cervical cancer screening? Clin Microbiol Infect. 2015;21(9):817-826.

ARHP. ARHP Patient Resources. http://www.arhp.org/publications-and-resources/patient-resources. Accessed November 30, 2015.

ASHA. HPV - American Sexual Health Association. http://www.ashasexualhealth.org/stdsstis/hpv/. Accessed December 14, 2015.

Atlanta GC for DC and P. Prevention of Genital HPV Infection and Sequelae: Report of an External Consultants Meeting - HPVSupplement99.pdf.; 1999. http://www.cdc.gov/std/hpv/HPVSupplement99.pdf.

Castellsagué X, Bosch FX, Muñoz N, et al. Male circumcision, penile human papillomavirus infection, and cervical cancer in female partners. N Engl J Med. 2002;346(15):1105-1112.

Centers for Disease Control and Prevention (CDC). Human papillomavirus-associated cancers - United States, 2004-2008. MMWR Morb Mortal Wkly Rep. 2012;61:258-261. http://www.ncbi.nlm.nih.gov/pubmed/22513527.

Centers for Disease Control and Prevention (CDC). How Many Cancers Are Linked with HPV Each Year? http://www.cdc.gov/cancer/hpv/statistics/cases.htm. Published 2014. Accessed December 1, 2015.

Centers for Disease Control and Prevention (CDC). ACIP GRADE Evidence Tables for Vaccine Recommendations | CDC. http://www.cdc.gov/vaccines/acip/recs/grade/table-refs.html. Published 2014. Accessed December 1, 2015.

Centers for Disease Control and Prevention (CDC). Advisory Committee on Immunization Practices (ACIP) October 2014 Meeting Minutes - min-2014-10.pdf. http://www.cdc.gov/vaccines/acip/meetings/downloads/min-archive/min-2014-10.pdf. Published 2014.

Centers for Disease Control and Prevention (CDC). STDs - HPV. http://www.cdc.gov/STD/HPV/. Published 2015. Accessed November 30, 2015.

Chase D, Goulder A, Zenhausern F, Monk B, Herbst-Kralovetz M. The vaginal and gastrointestinal microbiomes in gynecologic cancers: A review of applications in etiology, symptoms and treatment. Gynecol Oncol. 2015;138(1):190-200.

Chaturvedi AK, Engels EA, Pfeiffer RM, et al. Human papillomavirus and rising oropharyngeal cancer incidence in the United States. J Clin Oncol. 2011;29(32):4294-4301.

Chesson HW, Dunne EF, Hariri S, Markowitz LE. The estimated lifetime probability of acquiring human papillomavirus in the United States. Sex Transm Dis. 2014;41(11):660-664.

Chung CH, Bagheri A, D'Souza G. Epidemiology of oral human papillomavirus infection. Oral Oncol. 2014;50(5):364-369.

Colafrancesco S, Perricone C, Tomljenovic L, Shoenfeld Y. Human papilloma virus vaccine and primary ovarian failure: another facet of the autoimmune/inflammatory syndrome induced by adjuvants. Am J Reprod Immunol. 2013; 70:309-316.

Collins S, Mazloomzadeh S, Winter H, et al. High incidence of cervical human papillomavirus infection in women during their first sexual relationship. BJOG. 2002;109(1):96-98. http://www.ncbi.nlm.nih.gov/pubmed/11845815.

Cox JT, Castle PE, Behrens CM, Sharma A, Wright TC, Cuzick J. Comparison of cervical cancer screening strategies incorporating different combinations of cytology, HPV testing, and genotyping for HPV 16/18: results from the ATHENA HPV study. Am J Obstet Gynecol. 2013;208(3):184.e1-e184.e11.

Cuzick J. Gardasil 9 joins the fight against cervix cancer. Expert Rev Vaccines. 2015;14(8):1047-1049.

D. S, D. S, H.W. L, et al. American cancer society, american society for colposcopy and cervical pathology, and american society for clinical pathology screening guidelines for the prevention and early detection of cervical cancer. J Low Genit Tract Dis. 2012;16(3):175-204.

De Martel C, Ferlay J, Franceschi S, et al. Global burden of cancers attributable to infections in 2008: a review and synthetic analysis. Lancet Oncol. 2012;13(6):607-615.

De Sanjose S, Quint WG, Alemany L, Geraets DT, et al. Human papillomavirus genotype attribution in invasive cervical cancer: a retrospective cross-sectional worldwide study. Retrospective International Survey and HPV Time Trends Study Group. Lancet Oncol. 2010 Nov;11(11):1048-56. doi: 10.1016/S1470-2045(10)70230-8. Epub 2010 Oct 15

De Sanjosé S, Alemany L, Ordi J, Tous S, Alejo M, Bigby SM, Joura EA.

De Sanjosé S, Bruni L, Alemany L. HPV in genital cancers (at the exception of cervical cancer) and anal cancers. Presse Med. 2014 Oct 30; 43(12P2):e423-e428. doi: 10.1016/j.lpm.2014.10.001.

De Sanjosé S, Ibáñez R, Rodríguez-Salés V, Peris M, Roura E, Diaz M, Torné A, Costa D, Canet Y, Falguera G, Alejo M, Espinàs JA, Bosch FX. Screening of cervical cancer in Catalonia 2006-2012. Ecancermedicalscience. 2015 Apr 29; 9:532. doi: 10.3332/ecancer.2015.532. eCollection 2015.

Doorbar J, Egawa N, Griffin H, Kranjec C, Murakami I. Human papillomavirus molecular biology and disease association. Rev Med Virol. 2015;25 Suppl 1:2-23.

Eur J. Cancer. Worldwide human papillomavirus genotype attribution in over 2000 cases of intraepithelial and invasive lesions of the vulva. 2013 Nov;49(16):3450-61. doi: 10.1016/j.ejca.2013.06.033. Epub 2013 Jul 22.

Food and Drug Administration. FDA News Release: FDA approves Gardasil 9 for prevention of certain cancers caused by five additional types of HPV. Press Release. http://www.fda.gov/NewsEvents/Newsroom/PressAnnouncements/ucm426485.htm. Published 2014.

Forman D, de Martel C, Lacey CJ, et al. Global burden of human papillomavirus and related diseases. Vaccine. 2012;30 Suppl 5:F12-F23.

G. K, O. V, P. K, E. P. Predictors and clinical implications of HPV reservoire districts for genital tract disease. Curr Pharm Des. 2013;19(8):1395-1400.

Gillison ML, Chaturvedi AK, Lowy DR. HPV prophylactic vaccines and the potential prevention of noncervical cancers in both men and women. Cancer. 2008;113(10 Suppl):3036-3046.

Hebnes JB, Olesen TB, Duun-Henriksen AK, Munk C, Norrild B, Kjaer SK. Prevalence of Genital Human Papillomavirus among Men in Europe: Systematic Review and Meta-Analysis. J Sex Med. 2014;11(11):2630-2644.

Herbeck J, Ondruš V, Dvořák V, Mortakis A. Atlas Kolposkopie G. Herbeck, J. Ondruš, V. Dvořák, A. Mortakis - Portaro - Bibliothekskatalog.; 2010.

Herrero R, González P, Markowitz LE. Present status of human papillomavirus vaccine development and implementation. Lancet Oncol. 2015;16(5):e206-e216.

Hildesheim A, Herrero R, Wacholder S, et al. Effect of human papillomavirus 16/18 L1 viruslike particle vaccine among young women with preexisting infection: a randomized trial. JAMA. 2007;298(7):743-753.

IARC. Human Papillomaviruses. Vol 90.; 2007. http://monographs.iarc.fr/ENG/Monographs/vol90/mono90-6.pdf.

Jemal A, Simard EP, Dorell C, et al. Annual Report to the Nation on the Status of Cancer, 1975-2009, featuring the burden and trends in human papillomavirus(HPV)-associated cancers and HPV vaccination coverage levels. J Natl Cancer Inst. 2013;105(3):175-201.

Joura EA, Giuliano AR, Iversen O-E, et al. A 9-Valent HPV Vaccine against Infection and Intraepithelial Neoplasia in Women. N Engl J Med. 2015;372(8):711-723.

Karakitsos P, Chrelias C, Pouliakis A, et al. Identification of women for referral to colposcopy by neural networks: a preliminary study based on LBC and molecular biomarkers. J Biomed Biotechnol. 2012;2012:303192.

Kyrgiou M, Mitra A, Arbyn M, et al. Fertility and early pregnancy outcomes after treatment for cervical intraepithelial neoplasia: systematic review and meta-analysis. BMJ. 2014;349(oct28_1):g6192.

Lacey CJN, Lowndes CM, Shah K V. Burden and management of non-cancerous HPV-related conditions: HPV-6/11 disease. Vaccine. 2006;24(3):35-41.

Little DT, and Ward HR. Adolescent premature ovarian insufficiency following human papillomavirus vaccination: a case series seen in general practice. J Inv Med High Imp Case Rep. 2014; doi: 10.1177/2324709614556129, pp 1-12.

Lowy DR, Herrero R, Hildesheim A. Primary endpoints for future prophylactic human papillomavirus vaccine trials: towards infection and immunobridging. Lancet Oncol. 2015;16(5):e226-e233.

Lowy DR, Schiller JT. Reducing HPV-associated cancer globally. Cancer Prev Res (Phila). 2012;5(1):18-23.

Lu B, Wu Y, Nielson CM, et al. Factors associated with acquisition and clearance of human papillomavirus infection in a cohort of US men: a prospective study. J Infect Dis. 2009;199(3):362-371.

Management C, For G. ACOG Practice Bulletin Number 131: Screening for cervical cancer. Obstet Gynecol. 2012;120(5):1222-1238.

Markowitz LE, Dunne EF, Saraiya M, et al. Human papillomavirus vaccination: recommendations of the Advisory Committee on Immunization Practices (ACIP). MMWR Recomm Rep. 2014;63(RR-05):1-30.

Massad L., Einstein M., Huh W., et al. 2012 Updated Consensus Guidelines for the Management of Cervical Cancer Screening Test and Cancer Precursors. Am Soc Colposc Cerv Pathol. 2013;17(5):S1-S27.

Mayeaux E., Cox J. Modern Colposcopy Textbook and Atlas. Third Edition. 2012: 1-695.

McCredie M., Sharples K., Paul C., et al. Natural history of cervical neoplasia and risk of invasive cancer in women with cervical intraepithelial neoplasia 3: a retrospective cohort study. Lancet Oncol. 2008;9(5):425-434.

Meijer C., Snijders P. Cervical cancer in 2013: Screening comes of age and treatment progress continues. Nat Rev Clin Oncol. 2014;11(2):77-78.

Mirghani H., Amen F., Blanchard P., et al. Treatment de-escalation in HPV-positive oropharyngeal carcinoma: ongoing trials, critical issues and perspectives. Int J Cancer. 2015;136(7):1494-1503.

Mortakis A. Intraepithelial Neoplasia of the female lower genital tract. Colposcopic Atlas. Litsas Publications, Athens, Greece 1992.

Mortakis A. HPV infections of the Lower Genital Tract of Women. Litsas Publications, Athens, Greece, 1999.

Mortakis A. Women and HPV. Prevention of the infections and their sequelae. Litsas Publications, Athens, Greece, 2007.

Moyer V. Screening for Cervical Cancer: U.S. preventive services task force recommendation statement. Ann Intern Med. 2012;156(12):880-891.

Muñoz N, Bosch F., de Sanjosé S, et al. Epidemiologic classification of human papillomavirus types associated with cervical cancer. N Engl J Med. 2003;348(6):518-527.

Muñoz N, Castellsagué X, de González AB, Gissmann L. Chapter 1: HPV in the etiology of human cancer. Vaccine. 2006;24(SUPPL. 3):1-10.

Munro A., Cruickshank M. Impact of HPV immunization on the detection of cervical disease. Expert Rev Vaccines. 2014;13(4):0.

N.G. P, M. E. Human papillomavirus-associated head and neck cancer: Oncogenic mechanisms, epidemiology and clinical behaviour. Diagnostic Histopathol. 2015;21(2):49-64.

National Cancer Institute. Human Papillomavirus (HPV) Vaccines - National Cancer Institute. http://www.cancer.gov/about-cancer/causes-prevention/risk/

infectious-agents/hpv-vaccine-fact-sheet. Accessed November 30, 2015.

Paavonen J, Naud P, Salmerón J, et al. Efficacy of human papillomavirus (HPV)-16/18 AS04-adjuvanted vaccine against cervical infection and precancer caused by oncogenic HPV types (PATRICIA): final analysis of a double-blind, randomised study in young women. Lancet. 2009;374(9686):301-314.

Palefsky J. What your doctor may not tell you about HPV and Abnormal Pap Smears. Warner Books, New York 2002.

Paraskevaidis E, Arbyn M, Sotiriadis A, et al. The role of HPV DNA testing in the follow-up period after treatment for CIN: a systematic review of the literature. Cancer Treat Rev. 2004;30(2):205-211.

Research C for BE and. Approved Products - December 10, 2014 Approval Letter -GARDASIL 9. http://www.fda.gov/BiologicsBloodVaccines/Vaccines/ApprovedProducts/ucm426520.htm.

Rodolakis A, Thomakos N, Haidopoulos D, Antsaklis A. Management of relapsing cervical intraepithelial neoplasia. J Reprod Med. 2009;54(8):499-505.

Ronco G, Cuzick J, Pierotti P, et al. Accuracy of liquid based versus conventional cytology: overall results of new technologies for cervical cancer screening: randomised controlled trial. BMJ. 2007;335(7609):28.

S. H, E.R. U, S. S, et al. HPV type attribution in high-grade cervical lesions: Assessing the potential benefits of vaccines in a population-based evaluation in the United States. Cancer Epidemiol Biomarkers Prev. 2014;24(2):393-399.

S. H, Unger ER, M S, et al. Prevalence of genital human papillomavirus among females in the United States, the National Health And Nutrition Examination Survey, 2003-2006. J Infect Dis. 2011;204(4):566-573.

Saslow D, Solomon D, Lawson HW, et al. American Cancer Society, American Society for Colposcopy and Cervical Pathology, and American Society for Clinical Pathology screening guidelines for the prevention and early detection of cervical cancer. CA Cancer J Clin. 2012;62(3):147-172.

Satterwhite CL, Torrone E, Meites E, et al. Sexually transmitted infections among US women and men: prevalence and incidence estimates, 2008. Sex Transm Dis. 2013;40(3):187-193.

Saulle R, Semyonov L, Mannocci A, et al. Human papillomavirus and cancerous diseases of the head and neck: a systematic review and meta-analysis. Oral Dis. 2015;21(4):417-431.

Schiller JT, Castellsagué X, Garland SM. A review of clinical trials of human papillomavirus prophylactic vaccines. Vaccine. 2012;30 Suppl 5:F123-F138.

Shi R, Devarakonda S, Liu L, Taylor H, Mills G. Factors associated with genital human papillomavirus infection among adult females in the United States, NHANES 2007-2010. BMC Res Notes. 2014;7:544.

Soutter WP, Sasieni P, Panoskaltsis T. Long-term risk of invasive cervical cancer after treatment of squamous cervical intraepithelial neoplasia. Int J Cancer. 2006;118(8):2048-2055.

Stanley M a, Sudenga SL, Giuliano AR. Alternative dosage schedules with HPV virus-like particle vaccines. Expert Rev Vaccines. 2014;13(8):1027-1038.

Stillo M, Carrillo Santisteve P, Lopalco PL. Safety of human papillomavirus vaccines: a review. Expert Opin Drug Saf. 2015;14(5):697-712.

Suh DH, Lee K-H, Kim K, Kang S, Kim J-W. Major clinical research advances in gynecologic cancer in 2014. J Gynecol Oncol. 2015;26(2):156-167.

Urban D, Corry J, Rischin D. What is the best treatment for patients with human papillomavirus-positive and -negative oropharyngeal cancer? Cancer. 2014;120(10):1462-1470.

Vaccine Information Statement: HPV (Human Papillomavirus) Vaccine - Hpv_gardasil.pdf.; 2013. http://www.immunize.org/vis/hpv_gardasil.pdf. Accessed November 30, 2015.

Vichnin M, Bonanni P, Klein NP, Garland SM, Block SL, Kjaer SK, et. al. An overview of quadrivalent human papillomavirus vaccine safety – 2006 to 2015. Pediatr Inf Dis J. 2015; doi: 10.1097/INF.0000000000000793, pp 1-48.

Walboomers JMM, Jacobs M V., Manos MM, et al. Human papillomavirus is a necessary cause of invasive cervical cancer worldwide. J Pathol. 1999;189(1):12-19.

WHO. mono100B.pdf.; 2012. World Health Organization. http://monographs.iarc.fr/ENG/Monographs/vol100B/mono100B.pdf. Accessed December 1, 2015.

Winer RL. Genital Human Papillomavirus Infection: Incidence and Risk Factors in a Cohort of Female University Students. Am J Epidemiol. 2003;157(3):218-226.

Winer RL, Feng Q, Hughes JP, O'Reilly S, Kiviat NB, Koutsky LA. Risk of female human papillomavirus acquisition associated with first male sex partner. J Infect Dis. 2008;197(2):279-282.

Winer RL, Hughes JP, Feng Q, et al. Condom use and the risk of genital human papillomavirus infection in young women. N Engl J Med. 2006;354(25):2645-2654.

GLOSSARY

Adenocarcinoma of the cervix: A cancer consisting of tumor cells from the glandular epithelium (mucus-producing cells lining the endocervical canal).

AIN (Anal Intraepithelial Neoplasia): A tissue diagnosis in which abnormal squamous cells in the anus are found, which in time may progress to invasive cancer in a small percentage of patients.

AIS (Adenocarcinoma In Situ): Cancer cells in the glandular epithelium.

Anal cancer: Cancer of the epithelium lining the anal canal or the perianal region.

Anoscopy: The procedure in which a colposcope is used to examine the inside of the anus.

Anus: The end opening of the digestive tract.

ASCUS: Atypical Squamous Cells of Undetermined Significance. A mildly abnormal Pap smear that may or may not indicate a significant problem.

Biopsy: A sample of tissue. Also describes the act of removing a sample of tissue.

Carcinogenesis: The process by which normal cells are transformed into cancer cells.

Carcinogenic: Capable of contributing to the development of cancer; causing cancer.

Carcinoma In Situ: Malignant cancerous cells occupying the epithelium. They may progress to invasive cancer over time if left untreated.

CIN (Cervical Intraepithelial Neoplasia): Abnormal cells found in the epithelium that covers the surface of the cervix. CIN is usually caused by certain types of human papillomavirus (HPV) and may be discovered when a cervical biopsy is done. CIN is not cancer, but may become cancer and spread to nearby normal tissue. It is graded on a scale of 1 to 3, based on how abnormal the cells look under a microscope and how much of the cervical tissue is affected. For example, CIN 1 has slightly abnormal cells and is less likely to become cancer than CIN 2 or CIN 3. CIN 2 and CIN 3 are considered precancerous lesions.

Cervix: The "neck," or opening, of the uterus.

Chronic: Describes a condition of long duration.

Clinical infection: An active, visible infection; the most infectious expression of the HPV virus.

Colposcope: A microscope with a built-in light used for examining the vagina, cervix, and vulva.

Colposcopy: The procedure using a colposcope to examine the vagina, cervix, and vulva for suspicious lesions. It is sometimes accompanied by a biopsy of cervical tissue.

Columnar cells: The mucus-producing cells lining the endocervical canal.

Condylomata acuminata: Genital warts. (Condylomata - plural, Condyloma - singular). They are raised growths on the surface of the genitals caused by human papillomavirus (HPV) infection.

Conization: The excision of a conical portion of cervical tissue for curative and/or diagnostic purposes. A scalpel, a laser knife, or a thin wire loop heated by an electric current may be used to remove the tissue. The tissue is then checked under a microscope for signs of disease. Conization may be used to check for cervical cancer or to treat certain cervical conditions. Types of conization are LEEP (loop electrosurgical excision procedure) and cold knife conization (cold knife cone biopsy). Also called cone biopsy.

Cryotherapy: A procedure in which an extremely cold liquid or an instrument called a cryoprobe is used to freeze and destroy abnormal tissue. A cryoprobe is cooled with substances such as liquid nitrogen or liquid nitrous oxide. Cryotherapy may be used to treat warts and some conditions that may become cancer. Also called cryoablation and cryosurgery.

Curettage: The removal of tissue with a spoon-shaped instrument (called curette) to obtain a biopsy. Endocervical curettage is the scraping of the inside lining of the endocervical canal with a sharp curette.

Epithelial cells: The cells that line the internal and external surfaces of the body.

Hysterectomy: The removal of the uterus.

Imiquimod: A topical genital wart medication designed to stimulate local immunity and destroy warts.

Immune system: A complex network of cells, tissues, organs, and the substances they make that helps the body fight infections and other diseases. The immune system includes white blood cells and organs and tissues of the lymph system, such as the thymus, spleen, tonsils, lymph nodes, lymph vessels, and bone marrow.

Interferon: A naturally occurring molecule that has antiviral activity.

Intraepithelial Neoplasia: An area of abnormal intraepithelial cells. Possibly, a precancerous lesion.

Invasive cancer: The condition in which cancerous cells have spread from the surface of the tissue (epithelium) to tissue deeper in the organ (cervix, etc.) or to other parts of the body.

Larynx: The voice box.

Latent infection: The condition in which the virus is present but there are no signs of active infection. The patient is probably not infectious. Latent infections are also called dormant infections.

LEEP: Loop Electrodiathermy Excision Procedure. The excision of abnormal tissue by using an electrical loop.

Lesion: General term for any abnormal change in the structure of tissues due to disease.

LSIL: Low-grade squamous intraepithelial lesions. A diagnosis of mildly abnormal cells on a Pap smear.

Malignant: Another word for cancerous.

Metaplasia: Replacement of cells of one type by cells of another type, such as replacement of columnar cells by squamous cells.

Metastasis: The process by which cancerous tumors spread to tissues distant from the original cancer (from one part of the body to another). A tumor formed by cells that have spread is also called a "metastatic tumor" or a "metastasis." The metastatic tumor contains cells that are like those of the original (primary) tumor. The plural form of metastasis is metastases.

Metastasize: To spread by metastasis, by the bloodstream or through the lymph nodes.

Mucosal: Being of a mucous membrane, such as the moist skin surfaces of the mouth, vagina, or anus.

Neoplasia: Abnormal and uncontrolled cell growth resulting in a tumor.

Oncogenic: Capable of contributing to the development of cancer. Causing cancer.

GLOSSARY

Papilloma: A benign tumor growing from the epithelium of skin and mucous membranes, usually associated with HPV.

Pelvic examination: The procedure by which a physician examines the vulva, vagina, cervix, ovaries, and uterus.

Perinatal transmission: The transmission of a disease from mother to infant during childbirth.

Perineum: The area between the vulva and anus.

Podofillotoxin: A patient-applied therapy for genital warts that works by slowing down cell division. Also known as podofilox.

Premalignant: Precancerous.

Pubic area: The frontal genital area.

Punch biopsy: The procedure in which a sharp, round "punch" instrument removes a sample of skin for testing.

Recurrent: A condition that returns after treatment.

Scrotum: The sac of skin enclosing the testicles.

Shaft: The midsection of the penis.

Squamous cells: Flat, or scale-like, cells of the skin or epithelium.

Staging: The process used to determine how advanced a cancer is.

Stroma: The cells and connective tissues underneath skin layer.

Subclinical lesions: They cannot be seen during a simple clinical examination – they are invisible to the naked eye and cause no symptoms.

Trachea: The tube extending from the larynx to the bronchi; also called the windpipe.

Transformation zone: The area in which round columnar cells transform into the flatter squamous cells. The most common area of HPV infection, cervical or anal precancerous lesions, and cancer.

Transmission: The act of passing an infectious agent from one host to another.

Tumor: An overgrowth of abnormal cells.

Urethra: The canal carrying urine from the bladder to the outside of the body.

Urethral meatus: The opening of the urethra.

Uterus: The hollow, pear-shaped organ in a woman's pelvis. The uterus is where a fetus (unborn baby) develops and grows. Also called a womb.

Vagina: It is also called the birth canal (during birth, the baby passes through the vagina). Vagina is the sheath-like organ that goes from the uterus to the outside of the body.

Vaginectomy: The surgical removal of the vagina.

VAIN: Vaginal intraepithelial neoplasia. A tissue diagnosis in which abnormal squamous cells in the vagina are found. VAIN lesions may in time progress to invasive cancer in a small percentage of patients.

Vestibule: The space between the inner lips of the vulva, the opening of the vagina and urethra.

VIN: Vulvar Intraepithelial Neoplasia. A tissue diagnosis in which abnormal squamous cells in the vulva are found. VIN lesions in time may progress to invasive cancer.

Virus: An infectious agent consisting of a genome and protein coating that thrives and replicates only in living cells.

Vulva: The external female genital organs, including the clitoris, vaginal lips, and the opening to the vagina.

Warts: Benign growths on the epithelium of mucous membranes or skin caused by HPV. Genital warts are also named "condylomata acuminata," in medical books.

INDEX

Term	Pages
AIS	163
Anal cancer	211-213
Anal precancerous lesions	189-194
Cancer (what is)	196
Cervical cancer	200-205
Cervix of the uterus	97
CIN	162
Cold knife conization	175-176
Colposcopical biopsy	128-131
Colposcopy	124-128
Condoms and HPV infection	79
Condylomas	51
Cryotherapy of the cervix	180
Epithelium	50
Epithelium infected by HPV	102
Genital warts	133-153

Head and neck cancers	214-217
High-resolution anoscopy	193
HPV	
-and cancer	52, 195-217
-DNA	48
-Genital types	52
-Genotypes	48
-High risk types	55
-Infection	47
-Low risk types	54
-Oncogenic types	72
-test	109-110, 117-121
-transmission	69
-what is	48
HSIL	68, 159
Laser conization	167, 170, 177-178
LEEP	167, 170-175
LSIL	68
Metastasis	204
Mucosa	50
Papillomas	51
Pap test	105-116
Precancerous lesions on the cervix	157-182
Prevention (primary) with vaccination	80
Prevention (secondary)	80
Recurring respiratory papillomatosis	153-155

INDEX

Skin	49
Smoking and HPV	241-242
Subclinical HPV lesions	57, 134-136
Vaccines	83-95
Vaginal cancer	206-207
Vaginal precancerous lesions	184-186
Vulvar cancer	208-210
Vulvar precancerous lesions	187-189
Warts	61-63, 136-155

NOTES

Printed in Poland
by Amazon Fulfillment
Poland Sp. z o.o., Wrocław